# Peace for Your Mind
# Hope for Your Heart

## DR. TIM CLINTON
### With PAT SPRINGLE

CHARISMA
HOUSE

Visit the author's website at timclinton.com.

Library of Congress Cataloging-in-Publication Data:
An application to register this book for cataloging has been
submitted to the Library of Congress.
International Standard Book Number: 978-1-62999-921-0
E-book ISBN: 978-1-62999-922-7

20 21 22 23 24 — 987654321
Printed in the United States of America

*Anxiety does not empty tomorrow of its sorrows, but only empties today of its strength.*

—CHARLES SPURGEON

# CONTENTS

## Chapter 1

# A PANDEMIC OF FEAR
# AND ANXIETY

*My life has suddenly started to feel like it is spiraling out of control.... The uncertainty of what's ahead has become the most frightening thing, triggering fear and anxiety. The world has been brought to its knees by a tiny microorganism.... My goal is to do what's in my power to reduce the spread of the virus and to survive. I surrender what I can't control to chance, fate, or the mercy of God.*

—A New York resident, in response
to the COVID-19 pandemic

IT'S A WORD we've been hearing a lot lately, a word that invokes a sense of dread...fear...anxiety. It alerts us to a severe, widespread, and growing danger over which we have little if any control. As the pandemic has spread, so has the national level of anxiety. Every day we tune in to the news and watch the number of cases, deaths, and "hot spots" rise. It's consuming and alarming. Most are overdosing on what has been happening, and it's driving us insane. My wife, Julie, looked at me while watching a press briefing and said, "I've got to turn this off for a while. It's making me crazy!"

We've had other recent national crises, of course, but none that seem to have had the same degree of devastation that this pandemic has created. Perhaps the best comparison we have is the Great Depression that began in 1929. We've heard grandparents or great-grandparents reminisce about the ravages of unemployment, food shortages, the year dry winds blew 850 million tons of soil of the southern plains to the east coast, and a pervasive sense of hopelessness, but that seems like ancient history.

However, most of us remember the Y2K (year 2000) scare. During the late 1990s, computer programmers realized that their shortcut of using only the last two digits of the year when storing a date might create problems when every computer in the world changed from year "99" to year "00." What would happen? Would the computer date register as 1900? Or not at all? The cover of *Time* magazine early in 1999 asked, "The End of the World!?!" and prompted a year of rampant speculation.

Computer programmers got a good jump on resolving the Y2K issue, but as the millennium approached, public anxiety created a growing sense of alarm. People feared that prisons might erroneously release dangerous criminals; malfunctioning traffic lights could cause a plague of car accidents; planes might fall out of the sky; nuclear power plants could go offline and create dozens of Chernobyls. People began to hoard cash, fearing that bank records might become unreliable. But despite all the worst-case scenarios, the year 2000 rolled in with only a few minor technological glitches.

Less than two years later, however, the United States suffered a much more severe and lasting crisis. The September 11 attacks on the Pentagon and World Trade Center towers in 2001 came without warning, and the public instantly realized that life as they had known it would never be the same.

Although it didn't take too long to figure out who was behind the attacks and what response was appropriate, the anxiety level that spiked that day has stayed with us. In the aftermath most of us were convinced that our American resolve would see us through the crisis eventually. Still, we had seen what could happen if we drop our guard, so we started viewing other people with suspicion. Even today, every time we go through security checkpoints at airports or other places, we're subconsciously reminded of potential danger.

But now, the COVID-19 pandemic has left us reeling in unprecedented ways. Unlike the Y2K scare, we had little if any time to prepare to respond to this crisis. And unlike the 9-11 attacks, we lack sufficient facts to construct a quick and effective response. Early on, health experts were predicting that by the time the coronavirus runs its course, essentially everyone in America will personally know someone who died from it. While our scientists fervently work to create a vaccine and produce reliable testing that can be administered and evaluated quickly, our health-care workers struggle to try to keep the death toll from rising so rapidly.

*New York Times* columnist David Brooks recently asked readers to write in and describe their mental health during their time of isolation. He wrote that he was expecting "maybe some jaunty stories about families pulling together in a crisis."[1] But after receiving more than five thousand responses, he soberly reported that "everybody is suffering pervasive stress. But a lot of people are struggling with a misery that's much worse."[2] He included several examples in a couple of his columns.[3] One was used at the beginning of this chapter. Here are a few others:

- "I am normally a very positive person, outgoing, happy, energetic. Definitely a glass half-full. However, lately I cannot get through a day without tears, often sobs. I am terrified for myself and my family and everyone in the world. All the things I love to do, I'm now afraid to do."

- "I am overwhelmed some days with a sense of loss, particularly because I have not seen my grandchildren (three years old and ten months). My husband and I were their primary babysitters…We had them with us for ten hours most days of the week.…I miss their touch, their smell, their drool, their runny noses. We will miss Easter, my birthday and, in all likelihood, the baby's first birthday in May. I am angry at a force I cannot see, but more than anything, I am sad and aching to squeeze them again."

- "As a mother of three who has struggled with anxiety and depression before the coronavirus, this current situation has definitely magnified these issues and brought them to the surface.…My children have seen me cry and heard me scream more in these past few weeks than they have in their whole lives. I just pray they are young enough to not remember."

- "I'm struggling. I returned to my family's home earlier this year. I've placed myself back at the center of a highly dysfunctional household—generations of trauma, sexual abuse, alcoholism, depression and anxiety."

- "Our three grown children have all moved home. I am the glue that keeps everyone together, but I am feeling overwhelmed and weepy because I can't boost everyone up from their fears, disappointments and anxieties. I'm feeling useless, and that is depressing to me, in addition to my own fears about getting sick. After twenty-seven years of putting every family member's needs in front of my own, I am sure I need to see a therapist. I feel like I'm finally cracking and I don't even know why."

- "As a person with anxiety disorder I can only say that I am struggling to cope. Did I remove my gloves properly? Did I disinfect my groceries properly? Did I wash my hands well enough? I could go on indefinitely. People with anxiety disorders are always expecting the worst, and now that has come to pass. I am always terrified that I have slipped up somehow and will become ill and die."

Other respondents wrote of being "hog-tied to your unhappiness," of "invisible stress," and other consequences of pervasive anxiety. And at this writing the White House and the governors have a three-stage plan to take steps toward normal life, but it appears it will be at least a year before a vaccine or "herd immunity" completely stops the virus.[4] In the meantime we'll continue, at least in certain places, with required isolation and social distancing.

## THE REAL PANDEMIC

From news reports and personal conversations it quickly became clear that fear and anxiety were spreading even faster than the virus itself. Anxiety has a propensity to accumulate and intensify. The course of ordinary life presents plenty of anxiety-inducing events: personal illness, deaths of friends and loved ones, family dysfunctions, work conflicts, financial burdens, and so forth. Now, as a worldwide, potentially deadly disease spreads, we don't replace one source of fear with another. Our new anxieties simply pile on to the previous ones.

One reason the COVID-19 crisis is being compared to the Great Depression is the fact that it attacks our sense of what's normal at so many different levels. The *physical consequences* are the most evident. Coronavirus is a new disease, so at the beginning, no one had immunity. It affects breathing, so it is especially dangerous to those with preexisting conditions (asthma, COPD, weight problems, high blood pressure, etc.).

The *isolation consequences* then become another major issue. Fear of contagion is bad enough, but those who suffer from some degree of depression depend on emotional attachments to get by. The truth is, all of us need connections with people. To be suddenly isolated from friends, therapists, regular church involvement, and other connections only intensifies the internal stress and anxiety in what has been dubbed "double depression." Other people have "touch deprivation"—a condition that weakens the body's immune system and worsens depression—that can only be improved through physical touch because human contact reduces a harmful stress hormone. These people are forced to choose between the risks of leaving the security of isolation and the danger of *not* doing something to remedy the imbalance in their body chemistry that fuels their depression. In still other cases people in isolation have become so afraid of contracting the virus and overwhelmed that, over time, suicide seems a preferable option.

As a result of imposed isolation, the *economic consequences* have added yet another level of anxiety. When the virus reached the United States, the nation's economy had experienced a decade-long growth streak with no significant declines and an average increase of 2 percent each year, and the stock market grew from a low of 6,547 in the Dow in early 2009 to a high of over 29,550 in February just before the coronavirus scare shattered confidence.[5] On that day, the future looked secure to most investors, but within months of the arrival of the virus, devastating losses in the stock market quickly obliterated years of gains. Unemployment statistics set new records. Although employees in essential services *had* to work, and some people were able to work from home, thousands of others were forced into isolation with no options for income. Even with the temporary payment reprieves offered by companies overseeing mortgages, credit cards, school loans, and government programs, the economic stress is severe.

At the time of this writing, we still have more questions than answers about how the coronavirus crisis will eventually

resolve. In the meantime, as we gradually meet the require-
ments to open the economy and, to some degree, continue to
observe stay-at-home orders and social distancing, the purpose of this book is to offer some helpful suggestions for how
we can minimize the anxiety levels that seem to keep growing.
I'm hoping to "flatten the curve" on the spread of anxiety.

## WHAT ANXIETY IS...AND ISN'T

Before we go too far, we need to clarify a few terms. Most people
tend to speak of *concern, worry, stress*, and *anxiety* as synonyms,
and usually that doesn't create any confusion. It's true that the
terms are closely related, and if you're struggling with one of
them, you're probably dealing with the others as well. But each
term has a distinct and discrete definition.

One definition of *worry* is "to think about problems or
unpleasant things that might happen in a way that makes you
feel unhappy and frightened."[6] It affects your thoughts. The
distinction of worry is that it never leaves your mind, but it
creates no physical response. It's helpful to distinguish between
*concern* and *worry*. Concern usually has beneficial results.
When we begin to confront a problem and make the effort to
wrap our brains around the issue, concern enables us to create
a plan and take action to resolve the problem. But worry is
concern that has overflowed its banks! When we worry, we
can't stop thinking about the problem—but it is seldom productive reflection. Our minds focus on the most negative "what
ifs," and our imaginations conjure up images of the worst that
can happen. We have difficulty shutting off thoughts of doom.

They play on a perpetual "repeat" cycle, often consuming our minds, hearts, energy, and time.

Like the difference between concern and worry, experts observe *constructive* and *destructive* forms of *stress*. A moderate amount of pressure brings out our creativity and produces energy to solve a problem. At work, at home, and at church, when we face responsibilities and deadlines—and especially new responsibilities and pressing deadlines—these moments often bring out the best in us. Constructive stress is what motivates doctors to save patients, writers to meet deadlines, students to complete major assignments, and employees to throw themselves into a boss' pet project. Then, when the stressful event is over, the person can breathe a sigh of relief and go back to normal life. Constructive stress also occurs when you're walking alone on a dark night and you hear a large animal in the bushes. Adrenaline kicks in, and you run like the wind or prepare to fight for your life. When the ordeal is over, your adrenaline level declines and the sense of urgency dissolves—but you have a great story to tell!

When our level of stress rises too high, it has a destructive effect: we can become exhausted, irritable, and confused. If it continues, either in severity or longevity, we can suffer the ravages of burnout, including debilitating physiological effects such as sweating, labored breathing, insomnia, an increased heart rate, heart problems, muscle tension, headaches, ulcers, and fatigue. In an article for Desiring God, Nancy Wilson observes:

> Burnout is what happens to us when we take on too much, and we simply hit the wall. Those duties you

once enjoyed have piled up way too high, and now you don't feel like carrying them anymore. They are heavy. They are hard. They are too many. And you are tired. The duties themselves have not changed— you have. The commitments and responsibilities are probably very good. Maybe you have been volunteering, teaching, homeschooling, counseling, hosting, helping, cooking, nursing, cleaning, organizing, car pooling, and then you are doing it all over again day after day. You can't see an end in sight and you feel absolutely fried. Spent. Worn out. Drained.[7]

*Anxiety* is a condition of prolonged and uncontrollable worry, stress, or fear. *Anxiety disorders* are even more problematic. *The Diagnostic and Statistical Manual of Mental Disorders* (DSM-5) of the American Psychiatric Association states:

> *Anxiety disorders* include disorders that share features of excessive fear and anxiety and related behavioral disturbances. *Fear* is the emotional response to real or perceived imminent threat, whereas *anxiety* is anticipation of future threat. Obviously, these two states overlap, but they also differ, with fear more associated with surges of autonomic arousal necessary for fight or flight, thoughts of immediate danger, and escape behaviors, and anxiety more often associated with muscle tension and vigilance in preparation for future danger and cautious or avoidant behaviors....*Panic attacks* feature prominently within the anxiety disorders as a particular type of fear response.[8]

For the person who is anxious, the emotional distress is out of proportion to the actual threat. When we suffer from anxiety, and especially an anxiety disorder, we pay a steep price in physical, emotional, spiritual, and relational aspects of our lives. The condition is described by Jeremy Engle, staff editor at The Learning Network, citing an article by Emma Pattee:

> "Anxiety in some ways is a response to a false alarm," said [Dr. Luana Marques, the president of the Anxiety and Depression Association of America], describing a situation, for example, in which you show up at work and somebody gives you an off look. You start to have all the physiology of a stress response because you're telling yourself that your boss is upset with you, or that your job might be at risk. The blood is flowing, the adrenaline is pumping, your body is in a state of fight or flight—but there is no predator in the bushes.[9]

Later in the book we'll look more closely at the dangers of letting anxiety get out of control. At this point, just be assured that having anxious thoughts is natural. As we'll see, even the strongest believers sometimes experience anxiety. For instance, Psalm 139 concludes with a prayer from the psalmist:

> Search me, God, and know my heart; test me and know my anxious thoughts. See if there is any offensive way in me, and lead me in the way everlasting.
> —PSALM 139:23–24

This psalm is traditionally credited to David, so think about that for a moment. This was the youngster who fought off bears and lions while tending sheep alone; who picked up a pocketful of stones and went running, unprotected, toward the giant Goliath; who later conquered the city of Jerusalem and defeated armies. His faith and courage can't be disputed, and yet here he asked God to know his anxious thoughts. If David wasn't reluctant to speak about his anxieties (and God included his admission in the Scriptures), we don't need to try to hide our anxious feelings. And like David, we're wise to share our anxious thoughts with our powerful, comforting, loving God.

## CHOOSING HOPE

Why is it so important to share our anxious thoughts with God? Because to be honest, we're not strong enough to handle them on our own. Especially now. We're currently undergoing a worldwide threat worse than anything most of us have seen in our lifetimes. Perhaps World War II was the last time so many of the world's citizens were focused on the same problem, but coronavirus is affecting scores of countries that never saw battles in that war. People are dying in numbers that are frightening to consider. It would be fruitless to provide statistics here, because they will be significantly worse by the time this book goes to print.

If ever there was a time to be honest about anxious thoughts and feelings, it's now, but in our coronavirus world we add one more element to worry, stress, and anxiety. We add *fear of the future*. People aren't just worried about their health and the economy, stressed out over rising unemployment, and anxious about finding a vaccine and then returning to some new kind of "normal." Those are valid concerns, to be sure, but even stronger is the fear of contracting the disease and leaving our families behind too soon, of losing friends and family members, of a national economic recession or depression that wipes out the financial security we thought we could count on, and not having a job to go back to when the virus is under control.

That's why we need to learn to take our anxious thoughts to God. We have very real and powerful concerns, but God is a real and powerful source of help. It's my intention to remind you, as I remind myself, of the abundant peace and hope that only God can provide during times like these. Our world has taken a turn for the worse, but our God hasn't changed at all. He's still sovereign and in control. Whatever we need, He can provide. He's still the source of every good and perfect gift (Jas. 1:17).

As I've watched the rapid spread of the virus, the resulting death statistics, the crashing economy, and the rising unemployment numbers inflicted by this pandemic, I've been reminded of Viktor Frankl's observations. Frankl was a prominent psychiatrist who was imprisoned in Auschwitz and other concentration camps during World War II. For three years he endured the cruelest, harshest conditions imaginable. However, in the midst of those atrocities, he also witnessed amazing and tender acts of kindness among the inmates, and he came to an extraordinary conclusion: regardless of the bleakness and brutality of the situations we face, we always have the freedom to choose our attitudes. Frankl writes:

> We who lived in concentration camps can remember the men who walked through the huts comforting others, giving away their last piece of bread. They

may have been few in number, but they offer sufficient proof that everything can be taken from a man
but one thing: the last of the human freedoms—to
choose one's attitude in any given set of circumstances, to choose one's own way.

And there were always choices to make. Every day,
every hour, offered the opportunity to make a decision, a decision which determined whether you would
or would not submit to those powers which threatened to rob you of your very self, your inner freedom;
which determined whether or not you would become
the plaything of circumstance, renouncing freedom
and dignity to become molded into the form of the
typical inmate.[10]

If a person can endure the horrors and indignities of a Nazi
concentration camp and still choose to not be broken and
defeated, we can make it through the anxiety and fear resulting
from this spreading pandemic. We can choose to pursue God
and experience His peace and hope. I'm not saying it will be
easy, but I hope to provide some practical suggestions to help
you escape any mental turmoil you're experiencing so you
will eventually arrive at the place of wisdom, hope, peace, and
strength.

In this book we'll examine science, psychology, physiology,
and other concepts to help us cope with anxiety, but the primary focus will be on the consistency of God's power, goodness, and love. To help you think through each of the issues,
you'll find some reflection questions at the end of every chapter.

Please think them through on your own, and then, if possible, discuss them with your spouse, kids, parents, and friends.

It's my prayer that as you continue reading, you'll increasingly sense God's peace for your mind and hope for your heart.

Think about it:

1. What is the worst crisis you've faced so far in your life? Has it been resolved yet? If so, what did you learn from it?

2. What is your greatest concern about the current COVID-19 crisis? How have your concerns affected your day-to-day life?

3. Think about your current life:
   - What are some things you tend to worry about?
   - What are some things that raise your level of stress?
   - What creates the most anxiety for you?
   - What are your deepest, darkest fears?

4. As you take your anxious thoughts to God, what requests do you want to make?

5. Do you think you can find peace and hope before the current pandemic is completely resolved? Explain your answer.

6. What questions do you have that you hope will be answered in this book?

*Chapter 2*

# BATTLING AN UNSEEN ENEMY

*We don't know how to social distance and stay sane, we
don't know how to stay socially connected but far apart. We
don't know what to tell our kids. We're anxious, we're uncer-
tain, we are...afraid....I know this from my life...from
twenty years of research, and 400,000 pieces of data. If
you don't name what you're feeling, if you don't own
the feelings, and feel them, they will eat you alive.[1]*

—BRENÉ BROWN

LUIS SERVED TWO tours in Afghanistan. He's been home
for a couple of years and resumed his life in a nearby town
with his wife and two young children. He holds a steady job,
and from all appearances, seems to have made a satisfactory
adjustment back into civilian life. But when he shares with me
every couple of weeks, he confesses that he continues to have
nightmares on a regular basis. He's home. He's fairly happy.
But his lingering PTSD is an ongoing concern for him.

In contrast, Sara's problems seem minor. She had asked
for some confidence-building tips because she had reluctantly
agreed to speak at a local civic organization and was scared to
death. The last time I spoke to her, she described herself as "on
edge." She was relieved that the recent weeks of imposed isolation had postponed her talk and had given her a temporary

reprieve, but she wished she "could just get it over with" and put it behind her.

Blake, on the other hand, was laughing on our last Zoom call. He suffers from agoraphobia and is never fully at ease outside of his home. He found it quite amusing that so many people are now complaining about their shelter-at-home orders. "Those whiners!" he chuckled. "Now everybody gets to see how I live." While masses of people were complaining about the boredom and monotony of not being able to get out, Blake was in his ideal setting.

If Luis, Sara, and Blake found themselves together on a church committee or a jury, they would probably not detect that they had much in common, but they share a common bond with almost 20 percent of adults in the United States: anxiety disorder. Luis' PTSD, Sara's fear of public speaking, and Blake's agoraphobia are three common examples. Others include separation anxiety, panic attacks, social anxiety disorder, and obsessive-compulsive disorder. But what distinguishes Luis, Sara, and Blake from many other adults with anxiety issues is that they're getting help. Although almost a third of US adults will experience an anxiety disorder at some point in their lives, only 37 percent of them will seek treatment.[2] It's a shame, because anxiety disorders are highly treatable.

## A NEW LOOK AT AN OLD THREAT

The Great Pandemic of 2020 has raised the level of anxiety in most of our lives, as well it should. In fact, if you're not anxious about something these days, you're probably not paying enough attention! Was that cough the first sign that I have contracted the virus? How are Mom and Dad doing on their own, in isolation? How can I pay these mounting bills if I don't get back to work soon? What kind of world are my children going to inherit?

We have plenty to be anxious about in the best of times, and even more as this pandemic plays out. As anxiety intensifies, people tend to go in one of three directions: quickly try to shake it off, obsess about it, or attempt to ignore it altogether.

Some people are much better than others about not letting anxiety lodge too long in their minds. We need to remember what we learned in the previous chapter: anxiety is frequently a false alarm. It generates intense concern, not over what is *certain* to happen, but rather over what *could* happen. Maybe. Possibly.

Indeed, if you're able to mentally bob and weave and land a few blows of your own before being pummeled by anxiety, that's a desirable option. Max Lucado advises this course of action in his own inimitable way: "Become a worry-slapper. Treat frets like mosquitoes. Do you procrastinate when a bloodsucking bug lights on your skin? 'I'll take care of it in a moment.' Of course you don't! You give the critter the slap it deserves. Be equally decisive with anxiety."[3]

However, not all anxiety is so easily swatted away. If it were, we wouldn't be seeing so many anxiety disorders. When a threat of some kind arises, many people's minds immediately rush to worst-case scenarios, and then they marinate in anxiety as they anticipate contracting the disease, or getting the divorce, or being rejected after such a great job interview, or whatever. Anxiety is no mosquito to them; it's a looming, formidable, unseen opponent.

At least both these first two groups confront their anxiety. The third group attempts to downplay the reality of the threat, trying to convince themselves it's nothing. They feel intense anxiety, but they don't want to deal with it at all. Yet anxiety can't be simply wished away: ignoring it or denying it will eventually keep you up at night and give you ulcers. Research professor Brené Brown describes the dangers of what she calls "stockpiling hurt."

> In hundreds of interviews, people have recounted how they just "kept everything inside" until they couldn't sleep or eat or they became so anxious they couldn't focus at work or grew too depressed to do anything but stay in bed. Depression and anxiety are two of the body's first reactions to stockpiles of hurt. Of course, there are organic and biochemical reasons we experience clinical depression and debilitating anxiety—causes over which we have no control—but unrecognized pain and unprocessed hurt can also lead there.[4]

Some people have found that a preferable alternative is to "make friends," so to speak, with their anxiety. Rather than pretending it's not there or trying to control it, they learn to live with it. Luis' PTSD and Blake's agoraphobia in this chapter's opening scenarios are two examples. The levels of anxiety they feel may never get down to zero, but with therapy and perhaps the proper medications, their anxious feelings become manageable. An even better example is Sara's fear of public speaking. Once she musters her courage and makes her public presentation, she will emerge a more confident person, perhaps not so reluctant to step out of her comfort zone next time. Don't forget: a certain level of fear is beneficial because it alerts us to surrounding dangers and motivates us to productive action.

Writer and long-time anxiety sufferer Laura Turner recently publicized her struggle to deal with constant feelings of anxiety. After years of attempting to eliminate them, she found a therapist who recommended that she see her unpleasant feelings as just that—*feelings*, not necessarily reality. Her therapist told her that negative feelings are inevitable and best dealt with by accepting them, learning from them, and then acting to accomplish her larger life goals. Laura writes:

> The idea that I could accept my anxiety—as opposed to trying to get rid of it—was revolutionary to me. And the way I do it—by recognizing it when I see it, saying something like "I accept this anxious thought," or perhaps even using my imagination to invite it in to stay for tea, and then telling it I need to move on to something else—has been more helpful than I could have even imagined....
>
> My anxiety certainly isn't gone, but its hold on me has significantly loosened since I discovered the idea of acceptance. It's so counterintuitive to allow in the thing that wounds me, but it turns out that befriending my fear has actually caused its voice to soften.[5]

## FACING YOUR FEARS

Taking that first step to make peace with anxiety can be quite intimidating. Anxiety is the adult version of the monster under the bed that many children fear. Kids are not 100 percent sure there's something there, but their suspicions are strong enough to arouse their fear. They could assuage their fears by taking a look for themselves, but who wants to take that chance? (At least kids are quick to ask their parents to take a peek and give them a different, more comforting perspective. Most of us need much stronger prompting to ask for help when we need it.)

In his popular course at the New School for Social Research in New York City, author and teacher Walter Anderson describes anxiety in a similar way:

> Have you ever noticed how your body reacts when you're anxious? Quickened pulse. Sweaty palms. Dry throat, just as if you were face-to-face with a creature who wanted to gobble you up for breakfast! Anxiety is so frustrating: all that energy, and nothing to do with it. You can't run or fight, because there's nothing to run from, nothing to fight. You sit with a knot in your stomach, anticipating danger.[6]

Anxiety is especially intimidating because you know it's there, but you can't get enough of a grip on it to put up a good fight. The good news is that no matter how powerful the enemy is—whether seen or unseen—you have the assistance of an even more powerful unseen support team.

I take comfort from the story of Elisha's servant in 2 Kings 6:8–23. The prophet Elisha had replaced Elijah and had proved to be just as powerful and influential. Israel was at war with the Arameans at the time, but the king of Aram was becoming increasingly frustrated. Every time he planned an attack, God told Elisha, Elisha told Israel's king, and Israel avoided the danger. It happened so often that the Aramean king thought he had an Israelite mole in his ranks, but his men convinced him that Elisha had supernatural knowledge of what was going on. The king determined that the first thing he had to do was capture Elisha, so he discovered the prophet's location and surrounded the city during the night.

The next morning when Elisha's servant looked out and saw a terrifying force of enemy horses and chariots, he skipped fear and anxiety and went straight to panic! But Elisha told him not to be afraid, and he prayed, "Open his eyes, LORD, so that he may see" (v. 17). When the servant looked out again, he saw the surrounding hills filled with horses and chariots of fire—a far more intimidating power than the Aramean army.

By that time the Arameans were approaching, so Elisha asked God to strike them with blindness. Elisha went out to them and said he would lead them to the man they were looking for. He led the blinded army straight to the king of Israel in Samaria, where God opened their eyes. Israel's king was eager to kill them on the spot, but Elisha wouldn't allow it. Instead he had a feast prepared for them and then sent them home, putting an end to their raids—for a while, at least.

We instinctively fear many of the things we see or feel. It's a protective instinct. But Elisha's servant learned that the fearful things we face won't appear as threatening if we acknowledge God's unseen power. Even an unseen enemy like anxiety or depression can become less problematic if we remember that we don't have to fight it in our own strength. God is always there for us, whether we see Him or not.

There's a New Testament version of this lesson. In his second letter to the Corinthians, Paul reminds them that suffering is part of life's experiences, but he assured them: "Therefore we do not lose heart. Though outwardly we are wasting away, yet inwardly we are being renewed day by day. For our light and momentary troubles are achieving for us an eternal glory that far outweighs them all. So we fix our eyes not on what is seen, but on what is unseen, since what is seen is temporary, but what is unseen is eternal" (2 Cor. 4:16–18).

We don't literally see our anxiety, but it's quite real. However, it's also temporary. In contrast, God's unseen power is eternal—it's available now, and always will be. Anxiety can be a tenacious enemy and may continue to be a problem, but it can't separate us from the love and confidence available to us through Christ. (See Romans 8:38–39.)

Later in the book we'll look at specific techniques you can use to work through anxiety—to break its grip on you so you can make progress toward greater hope and peace. Here, let me offer just one suggestion to get you started. One simple way to learn to minimize anxiety is to intentionally make yourself anxious about doing something, and then do it anyway. You should start with minor challenges, of course, because even they will seem scary or intimidating at first.

People have different anxiety triggers, so you need to choose something that makes *you* anxious. Think of some things you always go out of your way to avoid. Any of those would be a good starting point. Researchers say that even the smallest step outside your comfort zone can produce a surprising amount of anxiety. I believe it. I know a dozen people in my church who would probably rather crawl through a roomful of snakes and spiders than to have to sit in a different section of the sanctuary away from "their" seat one Sunday.

How about you? If you're an introvert who tends to avoid social gatherings, attend the next one anyway. Take a friend with you if you need to. Convince yourself to take an elevator ride if you normally take five flights of stairs to avoid any chance of ever getting stuck in one. Walk across that bridge that intimidates you. Teach that Sunday school class. Make the phone call. After you do whatever you determine to do, you'll see that your worst fears didn't happen. It's a reminder that anxiety often generates fear about something that probably isn't there or isn't going to happen. As you learn to face your small fears, you'll eventually become equipped to loosen the choke hold of anxiety created by pandemics and other huge concerns.

## DON'T JUST FRET THERE, DO SOMETHING!

People always find something to complain about. Not so long ago I heard two common complaints: "There's just not enough time in the day. If I had more time, I would..." People would usually conclude that sentence with a desire to get in better shape, devote more time to hobbies, read more, spend more time with family, and so on. The second complaint was similar: "Everybody's always wanting something from me. I wish people would just leave me alone. Man, what I wouldn't give to have a little time to myself!"

But I'm not hearing *those* complaints these days! Now people are complaining that they have too much time on their hands. They're bored. They want to go back to work. They're eating too much. They want life to be the way it used to be.

Suddenly, unexpectedly, we now find ourselves with more time and solitude than we know what to do with. How does that make you feel: Overjoyed or edgy? Serene or scared?

Considering the reason that we've all been driven into isolation, it's natural to feel anxious, worried, or fearful. But time and solitude are rare and precious gifts, so let's not miss the opportunities they provide.

To begin with, we should learn to value solitude—time alone with ourselves and with God. Henri Nouwen called solitude "the furnace of transformation."[7] And A. W. Tozer wrote, "We must show a new generation of nervous, almost frantic, Christians that power lies at the center of the life."[8] Believers now have an ideal opportunity to get closer to our loving God, which is the only way to keep this chaotic life in perspective. In solitude we're able to sense God's presence more certainly, to allow Him to reveal Himself to us as He did to Elisha's servant. If we aren't intentional about connecting with God during these solitary times, we run the danger of allowing solitude to turn into loneliness.

Similarly, we shouldn't allow anxiety to poison the abundance of free time we have now. Charles Spurgeon said that "Anxiety does not empty tomorrow of its sorrows, but only empties today of its strength."[9] Those of us who have an abundance of time on our hands need to put it to good use rather than fritter it away in fear and anxiety.

One more observation from Walter Anderson is relevant here: "Nothing quells anxiety faster than action."[10] The example Anderson uses is a student who is anxious about failing a test. Anderson suggests that studying for the test (taking action) is a much better use of time than worrying about it. If we can stop worrying so much about the future and use that time instead to *prepare* for the future, anxiety usually diminishes. The bottom line: get up and get moving.

The key to getting through worrisome times is to *do* something! We need to redirect our anxious minds toward productive ventures. Now that we have all this time, we even have the leisure of single-tasking for a change. Determine a worthwhile activity and then give it the time and attention it deserves. For example, you can get comfortable, sit peacefully, and really enjoy that book you've been wanting to read; pull out a favorite album and take some time to ponder the lyrics as you listen; spend extra time on your porch or at a window to take in the glory of nature as days go by and seasons change; ponder the mystery and wonder of God's great love for you. Get out those dominoes, go for a walk, and reconnect with your family.

Using our abundance of free time and solitude to strengthen our relationships with God will probably result in another worthwhile activity: service to others. I've found that the more time I spend with God, the more likely He is to remind me of the needs of other people I know. We can use our current free time to serve others, even in our solitude, reaching out to church family, friends, and neighbors through phone calls, social media, and video calls. But this may also be an ideal time to go old-school: to sit down and write some cards and letters. Most people still love to get real mail. (Grandparents, you may need an eight-year-old to show you how to operate your smartphone, but you can show him or her the power of a stamp.)

If the impact of the virus is extended and we endure a longer period of isolation, it may become more challenging to avoid being bored and grouchy. But if and when that happens, I suggest we remember that while we're looking for something else to binge-watch, our health-care workers don't have the luxury of boredom. They remain overworked, overstressed, and at risk. When I think of them, I realize I don't have any valid cause to complain.

For many of us this influx of available time is a once-in-a-lifetime opportunity. Don't miss it! Let's develop an appreciation for the benefits of free time and solitude so we'll continue to make the most of them—even after they're no longer imposed on us!

Think about it:

1. On a scale of 1 to 10, what would you say was the usual level of anxiety you felt prior to the recent pandemic? Had you ever tried to lower the number? If so, how?

2. How has the pandemic affected your anxiety level?

3. How do you tend to deal with anxiety? Explain your response.

_____ Quickly try to shake it off
_____ Dwell on it too much
_____ Attempt to ignore it
_____ Learn to live with it
_____ Other: _____

4. Has anything in this chapter encouraged you to try a new tactic to deal with your anxiety? If so, what?

5. What are some specific actions you can take to help keep your anxiety from accumulating?

## Chapter 3

# DON'T BELIEVE
# EVERYTHING YOU HEAR

*The way we talk about anxiety today, it is easy to believe
that all anxiety is inherently bad and forget that it's our natural response to threat or danger. We actually need anxiety
to survive; it prepares our body to respond appropriately in
the face of danger....Anxiety, though often painful, is an
important and adaptive part of the human experience.[1]*

—ANNABELLE PARR

EMMA, CLEARLY FEELING emotional pain and almost
ranting about the injustice of her situation, told me, "If I
had a broken arm and people saw my cast, they would understand. If I were in a wheelchair, they would be sympathetic
and cut me some slack. But my problems are in my head. They
aren't visible. When people look at me, all they see is a pathetic,
forgetful, pitiful woman. It's like anxiety and depression aren't
legitimate problems."

"Do you get a lot of insensitive comments?" I asked.

Emma looked a bit sheepish. "Well, no," she admitted. "But
I know what they're thinking."

Emma may have come to some exaggerated conclusions
about the number of people who think she's just making up
her problems, but she's right that for far too long, people—and
especially believers—have attached a stigma to mental health.

In this chapter I want to address several false presumptions about anxiety and related issues. I hope we can put an end to many of the damaging myths that continue to circulate.

### Myth #1: Anxiety is the result of sin or lack of faith.

It was a big day for Eli, a corporate executive. He was scheduled to make a crucial presentation to the stockholders, one that he considered essential to the existence of the company. But he was aware that he was massively outnumbered. All the other executives had established a power bloc to oppose his radical idea, and they were confident the stockholders would see things their way. In addition, they were making their case first. Eli had no allies today; he was on his own.

His detractors spent the entire morning making their pitch. They were persistent, repetitive, loud, and even frenzied at times. They used every method they could think of to show the stockholders the soundness of their perspective, but it seemed that the harder they tried to sway the crowd, the less persuasive they became. Finally by the middle of the afternoon they were exhausted and out of ideas, so they yielded the floor.

Eli was ready. He knew the stockholders were tired by then, so he didn't waste any words. He spoke with unquestionable authority as he gave a brief demonstration to show them what needed to be done, and they were astounded at how evident it was that he knew what he was talking about. They took a vote right away, supporting Eli's proposal. Seemingly against all odds, he had done it!

Unfortunately the story didn't end there. As it turned out, the CEO and COO of the organization weren't fans of Eli. They disagreed with what he had done to "their" company and were determined to reverse the results of the vote. In fact, they made their displeasure clear with some not-so-subtle threats to the point that Eli even began to fear for his life. He immediately rushed to his car and drove for an entire day before he stopped for the night to reflect on what he should do next. He was feeling alone and vulnerable, and that night he asked God what any of us would in that situation: "What's going on?"

If you haven't guessed by now, Eli's story is actually that of the prophet Elijah, put in a modern setting. (See 1 Kings 18–19.) I can think of no better biblical example to disprove this first myth that anxiety is a result of either a lack of faith or outright sin. The nation of Israel was being led into rampant idolatry by King Ahab and Queen Jezebel, so Elijah invited the people to assemble atop Mount Carmel, where he stood alone against 850 prophets of Baal and Asherah. The showdown on the mountain began with an embarrassing demonstration of the impotence of the false gods. Despite their best efforts the prophets of Baal could not summon any divine response.

In contrast, Elijah began by dousing his offering with water not once, but three times. Then, immediately after he voiced a short prayer, fire from heaven fell to consume the sacrifice, the stones of the altar, and even the puddles of water. In response the people of Israel united with the cry, "The LORD—he is God!" (1 Kings 18:39).

Who would dare question the faith of Elijah—a faith that was consistent throughout his life? He was a mighty prophet to be sure, but he was also a human being. After Jezebel threatened to take his life within twenty-four hours, Elijah got scared, "ran for his life," and hid (1 Kings 19:1–3). If even Elijah, God's mighty prophet, wasn't immune from anxiety, why should any of us expect to be?

Elijah is by no means the only biblical example of someone who cratered under the power of anxiety. While traveling in unfamiliar territory, Abraham became so fearful of what might happen to him when some stranger noticed Sarah's great beauty that he willingly gave her up to local dignitaries—twice! (See Genesis 12:10–20; 20:1–18.) When King Saul was trying to take David's life, David hid among the Philistines, only to become "very much afraid" when they learned of his reputation of valor as a warrior. David even resorted to faking insanity to avoid a deadly confrontation (1 Sam. 21:10–15). Many other faithful and heroic biblical figures experienced anxiety, so don't let anyone tell you anxiety reflects an absence of faith.

### Myth #2: My feelings don't matter to God.

While we're thinking about Elijah's Mount Carmel experience, the latter part of that story helps to refute this second myth. Jezebel's death threat weighed heavily on the prophet, so much so that after going a day's journey into the wilderness, he even prayed for God to take his life. Instead God fed him. Two special meals—served by an angel, no less—sustained him for a forty-day journey to Mount Horeb (Sinai), where God told him to wait until He appeared to him. Elijah witnessed a great and powerful wind, an earthquake, and a fire—all impressive sights, to be sure. But it was only after those displays of power that God appeared, and when He did, He comforted Elijah with "a gentle whisper" (1 Kings 19:1–18).

By this time Elijah was confused, dejected, and in despair. He was also brutally honest: "I have been very zealous for the

Lᴏʀᴅ God Almighty. The Israelites have rejected your covenant, torn down your altars, and put your prophets to death with the sword. I am the only one left, and now they are trying to kill me too" (1 Kings 19:14).

How do you think God responded? With a pat on the back and soothing words? A World's Best Prophet trophy? A cookie and bowl of ice cream? No. God's first words were, "Go back the way you came" (v. 15). He didn't dismiss Elijah's feelings, but neither did He allow him to wallow in self-pity. Instead He gave Elijah three specific assignments. But before sending him back to work, God reassured Elijah that he was by no means the last of the faithful. Indeed, there were no fewer than seven thousand others who would join him in resisting idol worship and corrupt leadership.

And if you're still not convinced that God cares about your feelings, all you need to do is take a closer look at the life of Jesus. He put weighty theological discussions on hold to acknowledge the importance of the intrusive children who were running around (Matt. 19:13–14). He coaxed Zacchaeus out of the tree to share a meal with him (Luke 19:1–10). He made a point of confronting Peter's shame and forgiving him after Peter had broken his promise and denied Jesus three times (John 21:15–19). However, I think an even better example that shows God cares about our feelings is seen in the city of Cana at Jesus' first miracle.

The Jewish people had waited for centuries for their promised Messiah, one who would open the eyes of the blind, unstop the ears of the deaf, enable the lame to leap like a deer, and empower mute tongues to shout for joy (Isa. 35:5–6). It soon became clear (to some) that Jesus was that person. Indeed, when John the Baptist questioned Jesus' credentials (during an anxious period of his own), those miraculous deeds were the proofs Jesus listed (Matt. 11:2–5). So how did Jesus initiate this series of miracles? What was the first demonstration of His divine power? He turned 120 (possibly 180) gallons of water into wine.

You've heard the story from John 2:1–12. Jesus, His mother, and some of His disciples had been invited to a wedding where the unimaginable happened: the wedding party ran out of wine. In a culture so steeped in the importance of hospitality, this was an egregious breach of etiquette. The family would become a laughingstock, and the newlyweds might never live down the shame. Still, was this a significant enough matter for the Son of God to step in and display His amazing power for the first time? After all, there was no pressing physical need. Was soothing the young couple's anxiety reason enough for such a demonstration? It was for Jesus.

Jesus' action was prompted by His mother, but it wasn't a clear request. He could have easily declined to act. He had no reason to do anything, other than to alleviate the great anxiety of embarrassed hosts. But that was enough. Jesus recognized the hurt and embarrassment that would happen, and He acted. You can't tell me God doesn't care about my feelings—and yours.

Besides, God created us in His image, and the Scriptures give countless examples of the full range of God's emotions. He's the epitome of love and mercy. Jesus is the Prince of Peace. The Holy Spirit empowers believers with love, joy, peace, patience, and other qualities. From these and many other examples we see that God values our emotions, and just as much, He values our honesty about them.

### Myth #3: Christians shouldn't struggle with anxiety or depression. They should pray it away.

I know this myth still exists in some circles, but I've never understood why there's such a double standard between physical health and mental health. I've never heard people suggest that Christians shouldn't suffer with shingles or indigestion or diabetes. I've never heard anyone recommend praying away a broken leg. Treatment of physical illness and injury seems to be perfectly acceptable to the critics of mental health.

We don't mind calling a coronary event a heart attack, but it would be just as appropriate to call anxiety or depression a brain attack. The malfunction of the heart causes certain problems; the malfunction of the brain creates others. But both are physical, *biological* problems.

Some naïve critics seem to think that mental health issues are "all in your head," so to speak. The irony is, they are! But they are by no means imaginary, and they need to be treated as conscientiously as an appendix that threatens to rupture, a blood clot that is threatening to break loose, or an infected tooth that's causing intense pain and needs to come out. In fact, mental health issues may require more time and attention to diagnose and treat because they often include confusion on the part of the patient.

Another version of this myth is that believers shouldn't need to take antidepressants because faith in God should get us through any trying situation we face. I realize that some people's religious beliefs prohibit them from taking any kind of medicine for any kind of problem. I can appreciate that stand even though I don't agree with it. I also agree that some people are on medication that don't need to be. But what I'll never be able to understand are those who criticize believers for taking antidepressants or mood stabilizers who need them while they themselves are on meds for blood pressure regulation, cholesterol control, pain relief, and any other problem. It seems like a double standard to me.

Don't buy into this myth. If you're having ongoing struggles with anxiety, depression, or any other mental health issue, those problems are just as real—and just as treatable—as any other physical problem. You don't have to just accept it. God wants you to have hope and help, and the way that will happen for most people is finding the right doctor(s), medication(s), therapist(s), and other resources. All of those, of course, should be accompanied by prayer and attention to the promises of Scripture—but you don't need a spiritual guilt trip on top of everything else you're suffering.

### Myth #4: Talking about your mental health problems makes other people uncomfortable...or perhaps judgmental.

I saved this myth for last because it annoys me the most. I suspect the people who continue to propagate this myth are those who feel uncomfortable discussing their own painful feelings of anger, hurt, fear, or shame (such as the people I've previously mentioned who deal with anxiety by trying to ignore it). These people prefer to avoid the subject altogether rather than think about it too much...much less discuss it.

I talk with people all the time who struggle with mental health problems, and they're some of the most interesting, most courageous, and most authentic people I know. In our conversations I've discovered that many of them originally felt they might be judged by others if they were open about their mental issues, but those fears were soon dispelled when they started being honest and saw the wonderful support they received.

A friend told me about his wife's involvement in a Sunday morning service that focused on the women of the church. Women greeted people at the door, led the various parts of the liturgy, took the offering, and so forth. In lieu of the usual sermon, three women had agreed to speak for five minutes or so about how their faith made a difference in their lives. My friend's wife, Edna, was one of the speakers, but an especially reluctant one. I knew from previous discussions that his wife had been through some prolonged struggles with mental health issues, but I didn't know the details because he respected his wife's desire not to talk publicly about them.

He told me that despite Alta's initial reluctance, she realized the invitation to speak was perhaps a timely opportunity to finally open up about what she had been through. She struggled to determine exactly where to start or how much to share, yet she wanted the other women in the church to know how much she appreciated their support.

When Sunday came, she was told she would be the second of the three speakers. Alta fidgeted a bit as the first lady described several of the spiritual and relational difficulties she had worked through after spending most of her life in one denomination and eventually transferring to a different one. When she sat down, it was Alta's turn.

When my friend then started to describe his wife's talk, I could see the admiration in his eyes and hear it in his voice. He told me, "Alta had been nervous all week about what to say—particularly how much detail she should go into. She had shared her story with one or two of her church friends, who had been very supportive, but she had never been ready to make her problems public. Still, her recovery had gone well, and enough time had passed so that she and I were able to joke about it sometimes."

He paused for a moment and smiled before continuing. "When she stepped up to the podium, she just laid it all out there. She took a deep breath and told the congregation, 'About eight years ago, I went through a very difficult time. Our son was in the hospital having hip replacement surgery necessitated by his leukemia treatment. My mother had recently died. I was feeling a lot of stress at work and hadn't slept well in weeks. And one morning I just…I don't know what happened, but I lost touch with reality. My husband had to call an ambulance to get me to the hospital. After a few days I was eventually diagnosed with bipolar disorder.'"

My friend cleared his throat and looked up at me. "You could have heard a pin drop in that sanctuary," he said. "But she didn't stop there. She told them, 'I had three…they call them "episodes"…over the course of about three years. The first time, I was in the hospital for eleven days. The second time it took eleven weeks. Every time, after a recovery period when I thought I was getting better, I relapsed. But I finally found the right doctor and the right medications. I still have occasional memory issues, but I'm back to functioning almost like I used to. I wanted to share this with you because I'm so thankful for a loving husband and a supportive church like this one. When I was unable to exercise my faith, it was your faith that carried me through.'"

"She went on," my friend continued, "to acknowledge several of the specific ladies of the church who had taken her to lunch, sat with her in book club and Bible studies long before she was fully functioning, and in many other ways helped her find her way back into the community of faith. And when the church service was over, it took us half an hour to get out of there because so many people wanted to thank her and share their own stories. It was an amazing day."

It is not at all unusual for people with mental health problems to want to isolate themselves out of embarrassment or shame. It's often true that a few people will smugly judge those who are honest about their struggles, but the expectation that all people are going to look down on you or judge you is a myth. Fear can keep us in slavery to our secrets. The sooner you are willing to be honest with yourself and talk about your feelings with others, the sooner you can find healing and hope. Finding a safe person is a good place to start.

## UNTRUTH AND CONSEQUENCES

I've been calling these outrageous statements "myths," but let's use a more accurate term. They are outright lies. Jesus called Satan "a liar and the father of lies" (John 8:44), but the devil isn't limited to spiritual falsehoods. The myths we've just reviewed are untruths that, if you believe them, are effective in preventing you from finding the peace of Christ that's so abundant to those who honestly express their fears and feelings to Him.

In response to these myths, God has filled Scripture with many uplifting and encouraging truths. We will be looking at many of them in the chapters to come, but I want to focus on one at this point: you are invited to "cast all your anxiety on [God] because he cares for you" (1 Pet. 5:7).

Don't be confused; this is not the same as Myth #3's "praying away" your problems. When I see the word *cast*, I think of all my friends who are fly-fishing enthusiasts. They regularly pack up all their camping gear, prepare sack lunches, drive for hours to some remote creek or river, tie their favorite fly to their line, and cast the line out. If they don't hook a big trout on the first cast, do they then pack everything back up and go home? No way! They keep casting until they get what they came for.

I believe that's what God has in mind when He invites us to let Him handle our concerns, worries, and fears. Anxiety isn't quickly or easily expelled from our innermost thoughts. Someone has said, "Anxiety is a lot like a toddler. It never stops talking, tells you you're wrong about everything, and wakes you up at 3 a.m." But God is always eager for us to give Him our worries and ease our troubled minds, little by little. Keep casting your anxiety on Him until you get what you pray for. And like fly-fishing, the more you do it, the better you get at it.

Life is difficult enough without all the corrosive, toxic lies people propagate about mental health problems. If you truly want peace for your mind and hope for your heart, you'll see that these myths are roadblocks on the path to healing—for you or for someone you love. As you learn to cast them on God's broad shoulders and bask in the light of His truth, you'll discover God's blessings that you've been missing so far.

Think about it:

1. Have you heard any of the myths related in this chapter? If so, which one(s)? What was the look on the person's face and the tone of voice?

2. What other myths, lies, or questionable advice have you heard concerning anxiety, depression, or other mental health issues?

3. How do you feel about talking openly and honestly about your anxiety or other personal concerns? Do you have at least one person with whom you regularly share what you're truly feeling?

4. Why do you suppose so many biblical heroes who demonstrated great faith also suffered periods of anxiety, depression, and fear? And why do you think Scripture so often includes both their memorable triumphs and their personal struggles?

5. How good are you at casting your anxious thoughts on God? How do you think you might improve in the future?

## Chapter 4

# MAKING CONNECTIONS
# WITHOUT MAKING CONTACT

*People are complicated, and having touch of any sort requires*
*navigation, and I think that can be rewarding and I miss it.*
*I want to squeeze my friends and go on bad dates. Touch is*
*always complicated to me, so everything around the COVID-19*
*will just get thrown onto the anxiety list. And the relief and*
*joy will be added to the happy list. It has been a relief to*
*find out in this time how much I enjoy human company.*

—AN ANONYMOUS PERSON WAITING
OUT A PERIOD OF ISOLATION

MANY OF US have had occasions when, during a sweltering heat wave, the power goes out or something goes wrong with the HVAC system, and we tend to ask the same question: What in the world did people do before air-conditioning? My friends from the Deep South can relate stories of times when family members and neighbors used to start work at daybreak, take naps at midday, depend on fans placed in large, strategically designed windows, and stay outdoors as much as possible. Their large porches were neighborhood gathering places, and sometimes where they slept. Back when the heat drove people outside, they made frequent connections with one another.

After air-conditioning became affordable in the mid-1950s,

however, people started gravitating indoors. House designs changed, and the size of porches shrank. Some say that's when the South began to lose its charm, but it's also when Northerners started flocking to the area. If air-conditioning could get them through the wicked summer heat, the climate the rest of the year was preferable to the harsh winters they were accustomed to. People could tolerate sitting in theaters and churches in the summer. The Southern economy also flourished as numerous businesses moved south. With air-conditioning, chocolate wouldn't melt from the heat, paper wouldn't curl from the humidity, and other problems were remedied.

The South traded a decline in Southern hospitality for economic and municipal growth. Depending on whom you ask, air-conditioning was either the greatest invention since the wheel or the beginning of the end for distinctive southern culture. But one thing everybody agrees on is that Willis Haviland Carrier's invention was responsible for some drastic and lasting changes.

What I'm wondering is this: Will our current pandemic do to the church what air-conditioning did to the South? We've already seen the rapid spread of the virus usher in some startling changes. A few months ago it was unthinkable to envision an Easter when the nation's churches would be empty—when the pope didn't even conduct an Easter service at St. Peter's Square. Ordinary pastors became televangelists as many streamed their sermons. What other changes are in store?

No one knows how long the spread of the coronavirus will continue, or what necessary precautions will be established for years in the future. How long will it be before we again feel comfortable shaking hands or giving hugs? If we continue to wear masks, how do we know if the other person is smiling or scowling? Will the church eventually lose much of its character and power as people become more cautious and less accessible, or will it adapt and become stronger as a result?

In the meantime, how do we make connections with other people when we're not allowed to make contact?

## LOSING TOUCH

Air-conditioning was just one of many inventions that made life better but resulted in weakening personal connections. As more people stayed indoors on hot summer days, they had fewer "incidental" connections with next-door neighbors or strangers walking by.

Similarly the automobile provided new freedom and mobility, and people began to see employment opportunities in other cities. After learning of all the opportunities "out there," far fewer family members stayed in the communities where they were born and raised.

The internet was a new and wonderful source of information and communication, but it greatly reduced the need or desire to interact with other individuals "in person." And it has essentially killed off handwritten communication.

Even a gadget as simple and practical as the automatic garage door opener has taken its toll on personal interaction. Every day millions of people are able to leave and reenter their homes with no chance to speak to a neighbor. It's sad, if not tragic, that many of us no longer even know all our immediate neighbors. Is it true in your neighborhood?

Countless studies have been conducted and articles written to analyze how today's population is increasingly losing the personal touch. More recently, however, the articles are trending toward the problem of losing touch *literally*. People aren't touching one another as frequently as in times past, which is a problem because physical touch has all kinds of benefits that we're starting to miss.

Even before the pandemic the decline of human touch had been a growing concern. The rise of the internet was a major factor. It became quicker and easier to send an email down the hall to a coworker than to walk over and talk to her. And why ask a real person a question when you have Google at your fingertips?

On the heels of the internet came the smartphone tsunami, enabling us to carry the World Wide Web with us all day every day—with a phone and camera combined in a pocket-sized contraption. Soon it became common to see a couple in a restaurant on a date, both tapping away on their phones and not saying a word to one another. Add to the mix a rise in electronic gaming, and an addiction to various screens replaced human contact for many people—especially the younger generation.

Then, of course, we began to see the wave of famous people being exposed for sexual misconduct and losing high-profile positions as a result. It was a much-needed housecleaning to demonstrate that no one was above the law—and that everyone should show enough moral decency to treat members of the opposite gender with respect. Still, one unfortunate result was that people began to be hypersensitive about showing *any* affection (hugs, a kiss on the cheek, or even a brief hand on a shoulder) to someone who wasn't a family member or romantic interest. Doctors in England were instructed to avoid using hugs to comfort patients out of fear of potential lawsuits.[1] Teachers have become hesitant to touch students. Smartphone cameras are everywhere, and sometimes even the most innocent of actions can be misconstrued by onlookers unaware of the context, whose photos can wreck a reputation.

Now, in the pandemic, the potential power of touch is lost as millions of people are isolating themselves, whether voluntarily or by government order. Terms like *touch isolation* and *touch PTSD* are being coined to describe the phenomenon. We're hearing more about people in health-care facilities or hospital ICUs who are dying alone, with even friends and family prohibited from being there. It's hoped that the current fears and isolation strategies won't last long, but it's still so early in the discovery process that no one knows at this point. We've already been warned to expect a second wave of the virus after the first one winds down, so we try to bolster our faith and carry on as best we can.

## THE SCIENCE OF TOUCH

Touch is the first of our senses that we develop in the womb. Researchers have identified many benefits of touch—both psychological and physical—including better sleep, improved digestion, lower blood pressure, fewer and less-severe colds, and a stronger immune system.[2]

Skin is the body's largest organ, and it contains a variety of nerve endings that monitor constantly changing temperature, motions, and tactile interactions. Some receptors respond with that persistent itch you get after getting into poison ivy. Some respond to gentle strokes. Others react to pressure, pain, cold, heat, wind, or vibrations.

Francis McGlone is a leader in the field of affective touch and a professor of neuroscience at John Moores University in Liverpool. He warns: "We have demonised touch to a level at which it sparks off hysterical responses, it sparks off legislative processes, and this lack of touch is not good for mental health.... We seem to have been creating a touch-averse world. It's time to recover the social power of touch."[3]

Tiffany Field conducts similar studies at the University of Miami School of Medicine in the Touch Research Institute, which she founded. She says, "We know from the science of what goes on under the skin that when the skin is moved, pressure receptors are stimulated." When that happens, it "slows down heart rate, blood pressure and the release of cortisol," which gives people better control over their stress hormones. Being touched also increases the number of natural killer cells, "the frontline of the immune system. Serotonin increases. That's the body's natural antidepressant. It enables deeper sleep."[4]

One positive result of the COVID-19 pandemic is that more scientists are recognizing the need to know more about the science and meaning of touch, according to Victoria Abraira, an assistant professor at Rutgers University who specializes in the study of touch. She says: "This pandemic shows why touch should be studied in the same rigorous way as the other senses. For every 100 papers on vision, there is only one on touch. We need more scientists to study it, even if this is a nightmare experiment to have to go through. What I hope will come out of it is a sense of appreciation for touch, and the recognition that in studying it as a sense we can tap into the regions of the brain and how the brain rewires itself to be healthier and better socialized within humanity."[5]

Among the experiments that *have* been conducted are those that study what has been called "the Midas touch." Servers in restaurants have long been aware that a light touch on a patron's arm or shoulder usually results in a better tip. In one experiment to test this presumption, a researcher recruited a well-dressed young man to greet strangers in a park, shake their hands, and then leave. After he was gone, the researcher asked each person to rate the young man on a scale of 1 to 10 based on his dress and general appearance. The first test group of people rated him at a 5 or 6. But a second group evaluated him at an 8 or 9. Same words. Same dress. Same facial expressions. The only difference was that he greeted the people in the first group with a traditional one-hand handshake. With the second group, during the handshake he used his free hand to reach out and lightly grip the other person's forearm for a moment.[6] This one additional and unexpected connection through touch made a significant difference in the perception of being valued. Experiments like this one verify that people respond positively to touch, consciously or not.

When human touch is unavailable or not as abundant as we might wish, we may seek alternatives. The craving for touch helps explain a young child's fanatic attachment to a security blanket or stuffed animal. Manufacturers of sheets, clothes, and cosmetics spend millions in research and development to improve the tactile sensations of their products.

In the absence of other human contact during extended periods of isolation, it has been recommended that single people try to be more aware of any tactile contact to their skin, including walking barefoot across the floor, exercising, meditating, showering, washing hands, and anything else that stimulates the skin. Pets—even other people's pets—provide outlets for adults to have a nonthreatening touch sensation. These alternatives can be helpful, but they're poor substitutes for the real thing. The human body craves human touch.

One man in his fifties from New York described his efforts to keep up with his friends using technology. But despite his best efforts, he confesses to certain regrets.

> The one thing that can't be replicated is touch. I miss it. When I had a dog who loved to cuddle, I had a temp, a stand-in who filled the skin-to-skin gap in my life. But right now it's hugging a friend, the occasional accidental bumping of shoulders or brushing hands that I miss, as well—and maybe just as much—as intimate touch: a hand on a cheek, or two hands massaging my shoulders....
>
> Maybe one of the resets in my own life that this experience seems to do for me is making me realize how much I miss intimacy—and how much I've missed it for many years when it was potentially possible. The lockdown has made me appreciate physical human connection in a way I never had before.[7]

You too may be missing the human companionship you once took for granted. Let's turn our attention to what you can do in the meantime to maintain a mutually beneficial connection with those you care about, until you can be safely together again.

## START WITH YOURSELF

We emphasize loving God and loving others because Jesus combined those two priorities. He said "the greatest commandment" is to love God wholeheartedly, and the "second is like it," to "love your neighbor as yourself" (Matt. 22:34–40). But too many of us overlook the importance of taking care of ourselves. It's a mistake to ignore this practical advice. If an emergency occurs on a commercial airline flight and the oxygen masks drop down, passengers are instructed to secure their own mask before trying to help someone else. In most emergencies—especially extended ones like a spreading virus with little immunity in the early stages—you're little good to other people if you're falling apart. We care for them most effectively when we care for ourselves.

Start by considering your emotional state. We've looked at the importance of admitting and addressing anxiety, but the message is worth repeating here. As the nation and world continue to struggle against a new disease that's taking a heavy toll, how are you feeling? There's no shame in admitting feelings of anxiety, worry, and fear as you hear story after story of how COVID-19 has taken another person's life and devastated the livelihood of millions. These feelings should motivate you to take proper precautions for yourself and your loved ones. Don't be passive; don't let those emotions overwhelm you.

Turn to God to refresh your spirit, and keep casting your anxiety on Him, day by day. During your times of solitude, read Scripture to remind yourself of His promises, and listen for His reassuring voice. But take practical steps as well. Play some soothing music rather than listening to alarming news bulletins all day long. Open some windows and breathe in some fresh air as you look out at God's amazing creation and remind yourself that He's watching over the sparrows—and you and your family (Matt. 10:29).

What are you doing physically? After their first few weeks of isolation many of those who aren't working from home (and some who are) had already put on several pounds. Gyms are closed, and many of us have too much time on our hands, so it takes a conscious effort to keep from snacking all day long. Try to get some exercise even if it's just walking around the house or yard. Take on house cleaning, painting, or the gardening project you've been waiting for the right time to do. Determine your best options for staying active and focused on productive activities, and then do them! As you begin to restore a little peace and sense of normality and structure to your own life, you'll be better equipped to reach out to others.

## MAINTAINING RELATIONSHIPS

When you think about it, you may be surprised to realize how many people you used to see at work, church, Bible studies, clubs, sporting events, committee meetings, and around the neighborhood. Many of us frequently greet "the regulars" at coffee shops and restaurants, even if we don't know their names. It feels odd to suddenly lose all those contacts, and it's impossible to maintain connections with them all from the confines of home. Where do you even start to stay connected with the important people in your life? Who are the ones we should prioritize?

It appears there are several groups of people to consider: those who have lost their jobs and are in desperate need of food; those who are "essential" and must stay exposed as they serve in hospitals, nursing homes, farms, packing plants, and grocery stores; and those who are working from home, are still getting paid, and have relatively minor inconveniences. These three groups have very different needs and very different emotional responses. The first two are far more prone to anxiety than the last one.

Of course, put your family members at the top of your list. Once you've pulled yourself together, listen to their daily struggles and be an encouragement. Similarly, you will naturally check on your friends to share "war stories" about life in isolation, your hopes for a vaccine and economic relief, and your fears of rejoining the public after restrictions are lifted.

Also make it a priority to stay in touch with people you know who don't have much family support or many friends. If *you* think a few weeks or months of fear, uncertainty, and isolation has been difficult, think of those who were already in health-care facilities (many of which have been hot spots for the spread of the virus). A card or call can make a world of difference. And if you have young children, let them make the cards. Projects like this will be good for your family as well as each recipient.

Additionally, if you know anyone who is unable to escape repeated exposure to the virus (doctors, nurses, EMT workers, hospital aides, other health-care workers, grocery cashiers, merchants, etc.), put those people on your list. They're on the front lines of the battle against the spreading pandemic. Even during the first months we are hearing stories of health-care workers who, since they work around the virus all day long, haven't seen their children or spouses for weeks for fear of transmitting the disease to them. They've lacked necessary protective materials, and the stress they feel has been immense. If you know one of these workers personally, let him or her know of your appreciation, support, and prayers.

As you consider all the people you're missing, it might seem overwhelming to think about keeping up with them all. Don't even try. Most of them will probably be satisfied with a post on social media that lets them know you're OK. But in a time of crisis like this one, use your limited energy to connect with those who need you most. If you've had a running feud with a loved one, this is a great time for forgiveness and reconciliation. If a wayward child is aware of your great disappointment in him, this is the time to reassure him of your love. If parents or older relatives have become more fragile lately, be aware that they're in a higher risk category for the virus, and place them high on your priority list.

When you think methodically through all the people you might contact, it will become clear who should receive most of your time and attention. To effectively connect to those you want to help, you will probably need to postpone interaction with your less crucial relationships. Don't feel guilty. It's wise to temporarily let go of certain connections to strengthen the ones most important to you. It's definitely better than becoming overwhelmed trying to bolster everyone's spirits but your own. Then you'll be no good to anyone.

You have lots of options to maintain human connections with the people most important to you. Phone. Write. Email. Text. Skype. Zoom. Drive by their homes and wave. Send smoke signals. Do whatever works best for you to connect with those you care about. Let them know you're counting down the days until you can give them a loving embrace—and maybe a big bear hug. When the opportunity for human touch returns, you'll be ready!

Finally, trust the Holy Spirit to enable you to keep in touch with other believers. We remain one body even though, for a while, the individual members of the body may find themselves in isolation from one another. When you miss the oneness of the Spirit between you and fellow believers on surrounding pews, pray that the Spirit will enable you to feel that same connection with believers in surrounding neighborhoods, surrounding cities, or anywhere in the world.

Most churches livestream worship services every Sunday morning. The sanctuary is empty, but church members watch at the same time, realizing that although they don't see their fellow Christian brothers and sisters, they're still worshipping together. They are then able to post comments of encouragement to one another. Churches will need to adapt how they do things for a while, but God will always be with His people...regardless of the situation.

Pray with me that God will make us stronger people as we undergo the struggles and challenges that we face, and that His abundant blessings will keep us empowered and motivated as we do.

Think about it:

1. What have you found most difficult about social distancing, mask wearing, isolation, or any of the other inconveniences necessitated by this recent pandemic?

2. What, if any, experiences have you had with losing physical touch with other people? What have you learned from the experience?

3. What have you been doing so far to stay connected with people? Who are some additional people you might want to reach out to?

4. How has your spiritual life and growth been affected by the inability of churches to hold regular services? What disappointments have you felt? Have you had any positive results?

5. Do you continue to struggle with anxiety and/or fear? In what ways? Is your level of emotional distress going down? Rising? Or staying about the same?

*Chapter 5*

# FEEL IT

*Ignoring our emotions is turning our back on reality.
Listening to our emotions ushers us into reality. And reality
is where we meet God....Emotions are the language of
the soul. They are the cry that gives the heart a voice.*

—Peter Scazzero

Carla and Jonathan didn't know each other, but they had back-to-back appointments. Their stories were similar in some respects, but their responses were diametrically opposite. Both had stories of heartaches and broken dreams. Carla's childhood had been traumatic. Her father was verbally and physically abusive. He could be passive for days or even weeks, but she saw that he was a powder keg that only needed a match to blow up—and she never knew what that match might be. Her mother had learned to be emotionally distant from her dad, but she was also distant from Carla. Every day Carla's life was either full of drama or she waited for the match to light her dad's short fuse. Normal stresses of childhood and adolescence were intensified and multiplied by her family situation. To cope, Carla concluded that she needed to be stoic, strong, and not let anyone know what was going on in her heart.

After college Carla fell in love with Jose, and a year later they got married. They had two children, and soon she went back to work. For a couple of years she struggled to manage her career, her relationship with her husband, and their two rambunctious children, but it was too much for her. Her stoic mask had kept her anger and anxiety hidden for years, but now she blew like Mount St. Helens! She yelled at her husband in front of the kids, "I can't take it anymore! Don't you see that I'm doing the best I can?" She felt ashamed of her reaction and retreated into a shell. Her husband tried to talk to her about whatever had caused the explosion, but she refused. A week later it happened again, and again a few days after that. By the time Carla came to see me, she was more like her father than she wanted to admit: her husband and children never knew what match would light her short fuse and cause her to blow up in fury.

Jonathan also had a difficult childhood. His mother died when he was five years old, leaving his dad with three small children. His father was emotionally devastated by the loss of his beloved wife. He had a demanding job, and he poured himself into it. He asked his sister to take care of the kids until he got home from work each day. Jonathan was a sensitive boy, and he absorbed the pain in his family to a great extent. He couldn't articulate the hurt, fear, and uncertainty he felt, but it was very real. He couldn't talk to his dad about how he felt, and when he tried to talk to his aunt, she often told him, "Oh, you're fine. You have a loving dad and a happy life. Stop complaining." When he came for help, Jonathan wasn't exploding in anger; he was imploding in depression. He was frustrated and said, "I don't know what's wrong. I just don't have any energy, and I don't enjoy anything anymore. I have a hard time getting up and going to work, and when I'm home, I watch television all the time. Can you help me?"

## LIKE THE PLAGUE

Many of us avoid our emotions like the plague! We've spent a lifetime finding ways to bury the hurt, fear, anger, and shame, and we've become quite skilled at it. Some of us are sure that if we let our true feelings come to the surface, we couldn't control them. We believe they'd be like a squeezed tube of toothpaste: it's out, and there's no way to get it back in! Others try to convince themselves that "good Christians don't get angry, never feel hurt, and always rise above their shame."

When we don't have practice being honest about our feelings, we may not be able to distinguish between painful-but-healthy emotions and painful-and-destructive ones. The ones that are good and right include sorrow, grief, reasonable fear, and indignation at injustice; the ones that are destructive include rage, shame, bitterness, self-pity, and crippling fear. Because we feel threatened by any intense emotion, we've concluded that all of them should be avoided at all costs.

Many of us have developed elaborate (and fairly effective) ways to keep from feeling painful emotions:

- We minimize the pain: We say, "It wasn't really that bad." "It's no big deal." "No harm, no foul."

- We excuse the one who hurt us: We say, "Oh, she couldn't help it." "He didn't really mean what he said." "If you had his history, you'd act like that too."

- We rationalize: We say, "It's not my fault. My boss didn't make his directions clear." "I didn't really love him anyway."

- We deny reality: We say, "He doesn't have a drinking problem." "Why would you say Dad abused us? You're crazy. It never happened."

- We sublimate to redirect the pain to a more socially acceptable form: We say, "I live for my football team! I hope they *kill* State this weekend! No, I'm not angry at my mom at all."

The point is that many of us have become masters at avoiding the Pandora's box of the painful emotions we've hidden for many years.

## RAW EMOTIONS IN THE SCRIPTURES

As we look at the emotion of anxiety, we might ask, "Does God want us to feel anxious?" And we quickly answer, "No!" I think that's the wrong question. The right one is, "Does God want us to be honest about whatever we feel?" As we look at the Scriptures, we find the answer is a resounding "Yes!"

The wisdom literature in the Old Testament includes the books from Job to Ecclesiastes. We might assume they have similar themes, but actually they're quite different: Proverbs is a sunny day with a crystal clear view of right and wrong, the Psalms have sun with scattered showers (theologian Martin Marty observes that half of the psalms are "wintry"), Ecclesiastes is the long gloom of winter, and Job is a full-blown hurricane of trouble!

The psalmists are brutally honest about their perceptions and emotions, ranging from the highest heights of praise and thanksgiving to the lowest lows of despair and doubt. For instance, in only two verses David complains four times that God is taking way too long to answer his prayer.

> How long, LORD? Will you forget me forever? How long will you hide your face from me? How long must I wrestle with my thoughts and day after day have sorrow in my heart? How long will my enemy triumph over me?
>
> —PSALM 13:1–2

A few years ago, many churches sang a beautiful little song that began with the first verse of Psalm 42. When we read a little further, though, we see the context of the opening verse.

> As the deer pants for streams of water, so my soul pants for you, my God. My soul thirsts for God, for the living God. When can I go and meet with God? My tears have been my food day and night, while people say to me all day long, "Where is your God?" These things I remember as I pour out my soul: how I used to go to the house of God under the protection of the Mighty One with shouts of joy and praise among the festive throng.
>
> Why, my soul, are you downcast? Why so disturbed within me? Put your hope in God, for I will yet praise him, my Savior and my God.
>
> —PSALM 42:1–5

We might think, "Isn't it sweet that the deer pants for water and the writer pants for God?" No, it's not sweet at all! The deer is panting because it's dying of thirst, and the writer is panting because he's spiritually thirsty but God hasn't given him the water of love, hope, and peace. Instead, "My tears have been my food day and night." He's weeping. He's not just a little discouraged; he's in the pit of despair. People taunt him, "Where is your God?" And even his memories multiply his pain. He "used to go to the house of God...with shouts of joy and praise among the festive throng," but no more. He feels abandoned, hopeless, and desperate. He turns his prayer from God to talk directly to his heart: "Why, my soul, are you downcast? Why so disturbed within me?" He answers himself, "Put your hope in God" in the hope that He will eventually come through. No, this isn't a sweet little song. It's a desperate cry from the heart of someone who is on the brink of losing all hope.

When we read the story of David, we see plenty of times when his life was threatened—by King Saul, by foreign armies, by his own men, and even by his son. He was often on the run, just a step ahead of Saul's henchmen. Many of his psalms describe the terror he felt and his confidence in God. Is it possible to feel both of these emotions at the same time? Apparently it is.

> Be merciful to me, my God, for my enemies are in hot pursuit; all day long they press their attack. My adversaries pursue me all day long; in their pride many are attacking me.
>
> When I am afraid, I put my trust in you. In God,

whose word I praise—in God I trust and am not
afraid. What can mere mortals do to me?
—PSALM 56:1–4

David didn't voice this prayer when everything was calm
and his life was safe. He's recounting events in the present
tense. His enemies "are in hot pursuit" and "all day long they
press their attack." But in the middle of his fear—not after—he
chooses to trust in God.

In Psalm 73 the writer, Asaph, is really hacked off. He has
tried to follow God, be obedient to His commands, and live a
righteous life, but when he looks around, he sees wicked, selfish
people thriving while he suffers. He wants to scream, "It's not
fair!" For half the psalm he makes his case that God has let
him down, and he doesn't sugarcoat it at all. But at some point
God gave him insight into the bigger picture of God's justice,
and he realized he could trust God to do the right thing—
eventually, even if it appears that He's doing nothing now. He
reflects on the season of his rage.

When my heart was grieved and my spirit embittered,
I was senseless and ignorant; I was a brute beast
before you.
—PSALM 73:21–22

Does that sound like something we hear in church? No,
not very often. Asaph was completely honest with God. We
might paraphrase his outburst: "I was so angry and heartsick
that I was like a wild animal!" Have you ever felt anger that
intensely? If you have, you're in good company.

His honesty opened the door so he could experience God's wisdom (vv. 15–20) and a new, deeper sense of God's presence. In my opinion, one of the most beautiful statements of trust found in the Bible is Asaph's description of God "showing up" when he was in the deepest pit of anger and despair. After telling us he had been so upset that he acted like a wild animal, he takes us into a tender moment.

> Yet I am always with you; you hold me by my right hand. You guide me with your counsel, and afterward you will take me into glory. Whom have I in heaven but you? And earth has nothing I desire besides you. My flesh and my heart may fail, but God is the strength of my heart and my portion forever.
>
> —Psalm 73:23–26

Asaph tells us that when he was at his worst, God didn't condemn him or abandon him. God took his hand to comfort him, guide him, and reassure him. That's big! When Asaph was as angry and anxious as a person can be, the grace poured out on him filled his heart with love for God. I can almost hear him exclaim, "Whom have I in heaven but you? And earth has nothing I desire besides you." God met him in exquisite kindness, grace, comfort, and love.

Isn't that what we want? Isn't that the connection with God we long for? It only happened because Asaph was completely vulnerable in telling God that he believed He was unjust and uncaring. His honesty was the launching point for a far richer, deeper relationship with God.

In the New Testament, we usually look at the apostle Paul

as a rock of faith, but in one of his letters we get a glimpse of his emotional life. The believers in Corinth were a mess. They were jealous, immature, and missed the point of the gospel in more ways than we can count. Paul's first letter to them was a firm rebuke. Even the part in chapter 13 about love isn't what we normally think it is: Paul is saying, "You *aren't* patient, you *haven't been* kind, you're *terribly* jealous," and so on. But he begins his second letter with a very different tone. He has suffered, probably in a Roman dungeon for a long time, and the experience almost broke him.

> Praise be to the God and Father of our Lord Jesus Christ, the Father of compassion and the God of all comfort, who comforts us in all our troubles, so that we can comfort those in any trouble with the comfort we ourselves receive from God....
>
> We do not want you to be uninformed, brothers and sisters, about the troubles we experienced in the province of Asia. We were under great pressure, far beyond our ability to endure, so that we despaired of life itself. Indeed, we felt we had received the sentence of death.
>
> —2 Corinthians 1:3–4, 8–9

"Great pressure, far beyond our ability to endure" and "we despaired of life itself." In his letter to the Philippians, Paul had written that he didn't care if he lived or died: "To live is Christ and to die is gain" (Phil. 1:21). But here a lot of his confidence is gone, and he faces death with despair. Really? Paul? Yes, really. This tells me that no matter how strong, secure, and mature we are, we may come to a place where we feel shattered. At that moment we need to be honest about what we feel.

Let me give one more example, this time from the Gospels. Jesus predicted His death and resurrection many times, but when the moment approached, the weight of the world almost crushed Him. Matthew takes us to the scene.

> Then Jesus went with his disciples to a place called Gethsemane, and he said to them, "Sit here while I go over there and pray." He took Peter and the two sons of Zebedee along with him, and he began to be sorrowful and troubled. Then he said to them, "My soul is overwhelmed with sorrow to the point of death. Stay here and keep watch with me."
>
> Going a little farther, he fell with his face to the ground and prayed, "My Father, if it is possible, may this cup be taken from me. Yet not as I will, but as you will."
>
> —MATTHEW 26:36–39

Jesus had stood up to the sneering Pharisees again and again. They hated Him, and He knew it, but this was different. In the garden, Jesus looked into the abyss of hell and saw God's righteous judgment on the sin of every person who ever lived, and He was going to bear it all the next day. If anyone had reason to be "overwhelmed with sorrow to the point of death," it was Jesus. He pleaded with the Father to let the cup of divine wrath pass from Him, but He accepted His fate…because there was no other way to rescue us.

We could look at many other passages, like Gideon's dread,

Elijah's depression, and Peter's shame, but the point is clear: God invites us to take our raw emotions to Him. We aren't feeling anything unique, and He can handle our honesty.

## THE THRONE OF GRACE

The writer to the Hebrews offers us a challenge and a promise. First he reminds us that even if we try to bury our emotions and hide them from others, God knows, and God cares. He writes: "For the word of God is alive and active. Sharper than any double-edged sword, it penetrates even to dividing soul and spirit, joints and marrow; it judges the thoughts and attitudes of the heart. Nothing in all creation is hidden from God's sight. Everything is uncovered and laid bare before the eyes of him to whom we must give account" (Heb. 4:12–13). We don't do ourselves any favors by denying, minimizing, excusing, or rationalizing away our pain, fear, and anger. When we read the Bible (like we've been doing), God gives us eyes to see into "the thoughts and attitudes of the heart," which includes the full range of emotions. One of the statements about God's grace that I love the most is this: God knows the very worst about us, and He loves us still. We're safe in His arms. We can be honest with Him.

But the writer doesn't stop there. He reminds us that Jesus, the One who was honest with the Father in the garden, knows us intimately. His heart breaks when ours are broken; He's angry at the injustice we suffer; He knows what our shame feels like because He was cruelly mocked. The writer continues: "Therefore, since we have a great high priest who has ascended into heaven, Jesus the Son of God, let us hold firmly to the faith we profess. For we do not have a high priest who is unable to empathize with our weaknesses, but we have one who has been tempted in every way, just as we are—yet he did not sin. Let us then approach God's throne of grace with confidence, so that we may receive mercy and find grace to help us in our time of need" (Heb. 4:14–16).

Jesus empathizes because He's been there. He suffered and was tempted. He knows what it's like to feel abandoned and betrayed. He knows how it feels to pray earnestly and have the Father say no. Because He knows us so well, we can trust Him. He invites us to "approach God's throne of grace" with boldness because there we find what we desperately need: grace, mercy, peace, and hope. When? "In our time of need," when it feels like all hope is lost.

For many of us, that time is now.

## AUTHENTICITY

We can make opposite errors in how we handle our emotions. Some of us are too much in touch with our feelings, and they dominate every aspect of our lives. We have a hard time thinking because we feel so intensely. People have to walk on eggshells when they're near us because they don't know what will set us off. But many people are on the other end of the stick: we feel so uncomfortable with our emotions that we suppress them. The problem, of course, is that we can't be selective. It would be nice if we could suppress anger and leave joy unfiltered, but that's not the way the human heart works. When we suppress one, we suppress them all.

Yes, I know what you're thinking: "If I take the lid off and look inside the deep cavern of the emotions I've buried for many years, I'll come unglued! I can't handle it!" Some are sure their anger will cause an explosion. Others are confident their fears will be unleashed and haunt them for the rest of their lives. Still others have been hiding some dark secret, and they imagine the shame will overwhelm them.

The psalmists, Paul, and Jesus are telling you, "Watch me. I was completely honest, and it led to healing, joy, and peace." We might say, "Well, Jesus was murdered!" Yes, but again we look to the writer of Hebrews for insight: "Therefore, since we are surrounded by such a great cloud of witnesses, let us throw off everything that hinders and the sin that so easily entangles. And let us run with perseverance the race marked out for us, fixing our eyes on Jesus, the pioneer and perfecter of faith. For the joy set before him he endured the cross, scorning its shame, and sat down at the right hand of the throne of God. Consider him who endured such opposition from sinners, so that you will not grow weary and lose heart" (Heb. 12:1–3).

Jesus experienced great joy after He was honest with the Father about His dread of taking on the sins of the world. What was the joy that overcame the shame? It was you and me. He endured the most severe spiritual, emotional, and physical pain anyone has ever suffered, and He did it for a greater purpose: to rescue you and me. Part of what gives us hope as we're honest about our deepest feelings is that we can know that God has a greater purpose for us too. We can trust Him, and He'll turn ashes into beauty. In fact, our deepest pain—when God touches and heals it—becomes the source of our greatest impact on others. We'll have more insight, more compassion, and more spiritual power than we had when we were hiding and wearing masks to keep people from seeing what's really inside us.

But we would be foolish to try all this alone. We're wounded in relationships, and we're healed in relationships. To become more authentic, we need to find at least one authentic, safe person to be our friend and guide on the new path. It may be a counselor, a sponsor, a mentor, or a friend who has been down this road before us. This person will invite us to be increasingly honest about our anxiety, pain, and shame (because we'll continue to resist for a while), challenge us to see things through God's eyes, and experience the wonder of God's love more than ever before. How? Because we open the doors to places that we haven't let Him in before, and He graciously comes.

If you don't know a person who can come alongside you, ask God to show you. He or she isn't optional. It's unlikely that you'll make it without someone like this.

If you'd like to find a counselor or coach in your area, check out the Christian Care Connect resource on our website at aacc.net.

Think about it:

1. How does "stuffing" emotions lead to explosions or implosions?

2. What are some ways you've seen people try to block painful feelings?

3. Which have you used? How well did it (or they) work? Explain your answer.

4. Which of the examples of emotional honesty from the Scriptures touched you? What's your connection with that story?

5. Give your own definition of "emotional authenticity." Whom do you know who has it?

6. Do you have someone who will walk this path with you? If you do, are you being honest with him or her? If not, how will you find this person?

*Chapter 6*

# THINK IT

*A living faith is nothing else than a steadfast pursuit of God through all that disguises, disfigures, demolishes and seeks, so to speak, to abolish Him.*

—Jean-Pierre de Caussade

I don't want to think!" Richard was obviously annoyed with my suggestion that he take time to think about his response to his wife's cancer diagnosis. "Thinking is a waste of time. Just tell me what to do, and I'll do it." Richard's reaction is perfectly normal—when we're anxious, angry, or fearful, our natural inclination isn't to stop and think deeply; it's to do something—*anything*—to make it feel better! Oh, we want answers. We want them to be quick and complete, and we're very disappointed when we don't find answers like that.

Awful news can hit us like a freight train: a car accident, an unforeseen diagnosis, or the sudden death of someone we love. But sometimes we have more time for the reality of the heartache to set in: a difficult child has become a prodigal, financial setbacks, a worsening health problem, aging parents, the rolling news about a pandemic. Our gut instinct is always to shout, "Why? Why me? Why now? Why this?" Like Richard, many of us have a default mode of being unwilling or unable to think. The moment is too threatening, we're too afraid, and we don't have the mental scaffolding to come up with satisfying answers. We gravitate to leaders who confidently claim they have the answers, even if their answer is to blame someone or a group that they find inferior and threatening in some way.

When we try to get a sense of peace from refusing to think, we're setting ourselves up for more discouragement down the road. I believe God gives us peace as we think, but we need to focus on the right thoughts. It's easy to drift in one of two directions: either we're "just fine" because our thoughts are too superficial and rosy, or "the end of the world is near" because we get lost in the worst-case scenario. This type of "stinking thinking" can consume us.

Let me offer some suggestions to guide our thinking processes when we're facing difficulties and need God's peace and hope.

## 1. Grief is an essential part of gaining perspective.

As we saw in the last chapter, God invites us to be honest with ourselves and Him about our fear and pain. Americans aren't very good at grieving because we expect quick solutions and strategies to make the pain go away. But grief is an essential part of personal growth. We don't do ourselves any favors by minimizing what's true or catastrophizing—assuming the worst. Whatever our feelings are, we can express them to God without reservation. As we feel the pain and face the fear, we'll be open to God's perspective on the hardship. Grief doesn't happen instantly, or even quickly. God uses the process to unfold the truth of His love and give us confidence that He's in control.

## 2. Avoid knee-jerk blame.

Sometimes the connection between cause and effect is clear: God sent a storm and a great fish to correct the wayward prophet Jonah; God orchestrated events in Joseph's life to prevent famine from destroying his family; and God uses suffering to tenderize hearts and give us compassion to comfort others who are distressed, as we saw in Paul's letter to the Corinthians.

But when we ask why our loved one was severely injured in an accident, why our company downsized and let us go, or why God allowed a virus to kill tens of thousands and uproot the world's economy, we may not have clear answers. Theologian N. T. Wright gives direction for when we don't know the answer: "No doubt the usual silly suspects will tell us why God is doing this to us. A punishment? A warning?...Perhaps what we need more than either is to recover the biblical tradition of *lament*. Lament is what happens when people ask, 'Why?' and don't get an answer. It's where we get to when we move beyond our self-centered worry about our sins and failings and look more broadly at the suffering of the world."[1]

Perhaps the most eloquent answer is in the ancient Book of Job. In the story, we know about God's debate with Satan, but Job has no clue about it. He faces unimaginable losses: the death of his children, the death of his servants, the death of his livestock, and the death of his wife's support. For thirty-seven chapters of painful conversations as his "friends" blamed him for his troubles, Job wondered why God had sent such calamities. Finally God spoke, but He didn't give the answer Job was looking for. In the longest monologue by God in the Scriptures, He described His awesome power and majesty.

> Who is this that obscures my plans with words without knowledge? Brace yourself like a man; I will question you, and you shall answer me.
> Where were you when I laid the earth's foundation? Tell me, if you understand. Who marked off its dimensions? Surely you know! Who stretched a measuring line across it? On what were its footings set, or who laid its cornerstone—while the morning stars sang together and all the angels shouted for joy?
>
> —Job 38:2–7

And He was just getting started! We get the same kind of answer at the end of Romans 11. Paul spent three chapters describing the wonder of God's sovereignty, and he concluded with an effusion of praise.

> Oh, the depth of the riches of the wisdom and knowledge of God! How unsearchable his judgments, and his paths beyond tracing out! "Who has known the mind of the Lord? Or who has been his counselor?" "Who has ever given to God, that God should repay them?" For from him and through him and for him are all things. To him be the glory forever! Amen.
>
> —Romans 11:33–36

When we face heartaches and stresses, we may be able to connect the dots to the cause, but in many cases we can't. Still, we can have ultimate confidence that God is sovereign and good…and we can trust that His plans are good even when we can't see anything good happening around us.

### 3. The reason for suffering can't be that God doesn't love us.

One of the most common conclusions people draw during times of trouble is that God has abandoned them and doesn't love them, but this can't possibly be true. The cross demonstrates the enormity of God's love for us. The God of the universe sent His Son to take the judgment we deserve and pay the price we couldn't pay. In his beautiful description of salvation in Romans, Paul draws a powerful conclusion about the love of God: "What, then, shall we say in response to these things? If God is for us, who can be against us? He who did not spare his own Son, but gave him up for us all—how will he not also, along with him, graciously give us all things?" (Rom. 8:31–32). Jesus wept at the tomb of His friend Lazarus, He was grieved when John the Baptist was executed, and He wept over Jerusalem because He knew the city and its people would reject Him and be destroyed. And He paid the ultimate price to convince us of the enormity of His love.

His love never ends.

### 4. We have to fight for faith.

When we feel overwhelmed with anxiety, it's easy to slip into the twin poisons of our souls: bitterness and self-pity. We've been wronged, and we can't find any good reason for it. We've concluded (probably subconsciously) that God is no longer good, wise, and trustworthy, and we're really upset. Bitterness is delicious because it lets us pin blame on someone else, and our resentment gives us a shot of adrenaline that keeps us going. Self-pity is the other side of the coin. We *feel like* victims because we *are* victims, but reveling in our victimhood poisons our souls. Frederick Buechner explains why anger, bitterness, resentment, and self-pity are so attractive: "Of the Seven Deadly Sins, anger is possibly the most fun. To lick your wounds, to smack your lips over grievances long past, to roll over your tongue the prospect of bitter confrontations still to come, to savor to the last toothsome morsel both the pain you are given and the pain you are giving back—in many ways it is a feast fit for a king. The chief drawback is that what you are wolfing down is yourself. The skeleton at the feast is you!"[2]

The battle for truth, peace, and hope takes place in our minds. We need the discipline and tenacity to wrestle with our assumptions, keep the ones that line up with God's truth, and reject the rest. That was Paul's instruction to the Corinthians: "For though we live in the world, we do not wage war as the world does. The weapons we fight with are not the weapons of the world. On the contrary, they have divine power to demolish strongholds. We demolish arguments and every pretension that sets itself up against the knowledge of God, and we take captive every thought to make it obedient to Christ" (2 Cor. 10:3–5).

The strongholds are false assumptions, errors in thinking, and the whispers of the enemy. We don't tinker with them, and we don't tolerate them—we demolish them! How? By contrasting them with the love, forgiveness, power, and purpose we find in the Word of God. When our minds tell us we've been abandoned, we read that God considers us to be His treasures. When we're crushed with thoughts that "It's all my fault," we look at the truth about His compassion and forgiveness. When we feel utterly weak and helpless, we realize God the Holy Spirit lives inside us. And when we believe our lives are spinning out of control, we look at verses that assure us that God holds everything in His hands.

### 5. Have realistic expectations.

God hasn't promised a stress-free life. Jesus tells us to take up our cross and follow Him (Matt. 16:24). We share in the suffering of Christ. As fallen people in a fallen world, we live between "the already" and the "not yet." Many of God's promises—for forgiveness, the presence of the Spirit in us, and the hope of change—are already ours. But the ultimate promise of restoration—where sin, tears, and death are no more, and where we enjoy a face-to-face relationship with Jesus—are not ours yet.

St. Basil's faith was called "ambidextrous" because he held pleasures in one hand and heartaches in the other, believing God would use both to accomplish His divine purposes. In *Reaching for the Invisible God*, Philip Yancey explains this.

> Here is what ambidextrous, or "two-handed" faith means to me, in theory if not always in practice. I take "everything without exception" as God's action in the sense of asking what I can learn from it and praying for God to redeem it by improving me. I take nothing as God's action in the sense of judging God's character, for I have learned to accept my puny status as a creature—which includes a limited point of view

that obscures unseen forces in the present as well as a
future known only to God. The skeptic may insist this
unfairly lets God off the hook, but perhaps that's what
faith is: trusting God's goodness despite any apparent
evidence against it. As a soldier trusts his general's
orders; better, as a child trusts her loving parent.[3]

Although we face suffering as a result of living in a broken
world, we also have the full range of God's blessings. When
we're tempted to shake our fists at heaven, we need to culti-
vate "ambidextrous" faith, accepting everything as lessons in
the classroom of a wise and loving Teacher.

### 6. Find the right friends.

In this day of social media we're bombarded by the opin-
ions of millions of people. The sheer number of posts can give
weight to what we read, even if it's completely off base. I've made
a point of narrowing my input to a few trusted news sources
and a few wise friends. I look for outlets that have carefully
reasoned responses and offer multiple sides of an issue without
yelling or demanding that I agree. And I've found some wonderful people who are thoughtful, theologically astute, and
have the rare trait of wisdom that has been forged in the crucible of their own suffering. These people don't give superficial
answers to life's deepest questions...and sometimes they give
no advice at all. They're just there, offering their friendship and
love...and that's exactly what I need.

### 7. But someday...

The arc of the Bible's storyline is creation, fall, redemption,
and restoration. We're in the period of redemption now, but

the promise is that one day we'll live in the new heavens and new earth. What difference does this promise make to those who struggle with fear, anxiety, and depression? A lot! If I looked in my wallet and saw that I had only a few dollars and the bills were piling up, it would give me incredible relief if a bank called with the news that an unknown relative had died and left me a billion dollars, and it would be deposited in my account tomorrow! Today the presence of the Spirit is a "down payment," but tomorrow we'll share in His fullness when we're with God in His city. That's our hope. That's our certainty.

What will it be like? The biblical authors had a hard time describing something so wonderful, but in C. S. Lewis' sermon called "The Weight of Glory," delivered during a bleak time in World War II, he crystallizes the Scriptures' teaching. Lewis says that five things will be true of us in the new heavens and new earth: we'll be with Jesus, we'll be like Jesus, we'll celebrate at a family feast again and again, God will delight in us as His children (which is our sharing of God's glory), and we'll have roles to play in God's perfect kingdom.[4] When Lewis spoke this message, Britain had lost virtually every battle it had fought. The people needed a message of hope, and Lewis told them about the glory that awaited them…and that awaits us.

Our confidence in our eternal destiny isn't a crutch to get us through hard times. It's far more than that. It's our bedrock of hope that someday all will be right, all will be well, and all will be beautiful.

### 8. Think about Jesus.

While reading this book, some of you have been thinking again and again of Paul's admonition in his letter to the

Philippians: "Do not be anxious about anything, but in every situation, by prayer and petition, with thanksgiving, present your requests to God. And the peace of God, which transcends all understanding, will guard your hearts and your minds in Christ Jesus" (Phil. 4:6–7). But this can't mean that the emotion of anxiety is a sin because, as we saw in the last chapter, the psalmists, Paul, and even Jesus experienced tremendous emotional distress. And in fact, earlier in this letter Paul told them that his friend Epaphroditus had been so sick that he "almost died." When he survived, Paul said it was God's mercy on both of them, "to spare me sorrow upon sorrow" (Phil. 2:25–27).

The connection between the two chapters in Paul's letter is clear and strong. To address anxiety, Paul instructs them, "Finally, brothers and sisters, whatever is true, whatever is noble, whatever is right, whatever is pure, whatever is lovely, whatever is admirable—if anything is excellent or praiseworthy—think about such things. Whatever you have learned or received or heard from me, or seen in me—put it into practice. And the God of peace will be with you" (Phil. 4:8–9). We often read the Bible episodically, one verse or paragraph at a time, but in the church in Philippi the entire letter was read, probably quite often. This enabled the people to connect the dots back to chapter 2.

Jesus is true, noble, right, pure, lovely, admirable, excellent, and praiseworthy. This is how Paul had described Jesus earlier in the letter.

> Who, being in very nature God, did not consider equality with God something to be used to his own advantage; rather, he made himself nothing by taking

the very nature of a servant, being made in human likeness, and being found in appearance as a man, he humbled himself by becoming obedient to death— even death on a cross!

Therefore God exalted him to the highest place and gave him the name that is above every name, that at the name of Jesus every knee should bow, in heaven and on earth and under the earth, and every tongue acknowledge that Jesus Christ is Lord, to the glory of God the Father.

—PHILIPPIANS 2:6–11

When I'm anxious, my thoughts naturally dwell on my problems, and I can spiral down into despair. But over the years I've learned to shift my focus from my problems to my Savior. If anyone understands, He does. If anyone cares, He does. If anyone suffered unjustly but still trusted the Father, He did. He is more than my example; He's "the author and finisher of our faith" (Heb. 12:2, KJV).

As we look at Jesus, we're amazed that He loves us so much that He was willing to suffer extreme injustice. In *Walking with God through Pain and Suffering*, Timothy Keller explains how Jesus uses our suffering to transform us.

Jesus lost all his glory so that we could be clothed in it. He was shut out so we could get access. He was bound, nailed, so that we could be free. He was cast out so we could approach. And Jesus took away the only kind of suffering that can really destroy you: that is being cast away from God. He took that so that now all suffering that comes into your life will only make you great. A lump of coal under pressure becomes a diamond. And the suffering of a person in Christ only turns you into somebody gorgeous.[5]

Please don't misunderstand: I'm not suggesting we should become masochists who delight in suffering. But I'm suggesting that if we learn to think rightly about the difficulties we face, we won't be crushed by them, we won't be distracted by them, and we won't let them ruin our relationships with God and the people around us. For many of us the learning curve is steep. We've grown up in the wealthiest nation on earth with astounding comforts and joys. People in other nations have had far more experience in learning to handle life's problems. Could it be our turn to learn?

Think about it:

1. Why do you imagine that some people simply don't want to think when they face hardships?

2. What are some examples of "knee-jerk blame" that come to mind?

3. Why do you think resentment and self-pity feel so right to so many people?

4. Is having "ambidextrous" faith attractive to you? Explain your answer.

5. Who is a wise, mature person who is your source of strength in times of trouble?

6. What is it about Jesus that we desperately need to think about?

## Chapter 7

# PRAY IT

*Our prayers may be awkward. Our attempts may be feeble.*
*But since the power of prayer is in the one who hears it and*
*not the one who says it, our prayers do make a difference.*

—MAX LUCADO, *HE STILL MOVES STONES*

FRANCINE HAD SCHEDULED several appointments, but she had canceled each one a few hours before we were to meet. When she called to ask to meet with me again, I wondered if I should double book because of her track record. This time, however, she didn't call to cancel. When she walked in, I could tell she was distressed.

I had barely introduced myself when she blurted out, "I've given up on God. I pray, but He doesn't answer. I plead, but He doesn't hear." She took a deep breath. It was obvious she felt ashamed of her conclusions about God. That's why she had missed so many appointments. But now she was desperate. "In the past few months, my life has been turned upside down. Before all of this, I had enough trouble trying to cope with two generations in our family. My mother is losing her memory, and she requires constant attention. She lives with us now, but we can't go on like this much longer. We've been paying for a home health nurse to come in three times a week, and that's gone on for the past year, but our savings have been depleted. The other major difficulty is with our son. He graduated from college, but he hasn't gotten a job. And now, with so many businesses shut down, there's very little hope of him getting one anytime soon." She paused for a second and then added, "Yes, he lives with us too. I'm exhausted, our finances are in shreds, I love my mother but I can't care for her, and I'd like to strangle my son."

I asked, "Francine, when you began, you talked about some struggles with prayer. Would you tell me more about that?"

She began to cry. "I've given up on God…I guess because He's given up on me. My husband feels the same way, but he won't admit it. He thinks it'll make him look weak. He's a pastor, and he wants to stay strong for the people in the church. Can you help me?"

## DIG DEEPER

In parts of Texas that get little rain, farmers have some of the biggest cotton fields in the nation. Irrigation has enabled them to draw an enormous amount of water from underground aquifers—so much, in fact, that before-and-after pictures show the land has sunk thirty feet in some areas. But there's a problem: the vast fields of cotton are threatened because the water is running out. The farmers have a solution, though. It's to dig deeper to tap into resources not previously available. That's a metaphor of prayer during times of emotional, financial, and spiritual drought. We have to dig deeper.

God invites us to come to Him with our requests—big or small, clear or not. When we're anxious, we pray for relief, for God to change the circumstances that cause us such worry and heartache. There's absolutely nothing wrong with those prayers, but how do we respond when God doesn't give us the relief we long for? What happens when, if our situations are anything like Francine's, the health of those we love declines, our finances dwindle away, opportunities are lost, and our sense of hopelessness goes through the roof? When the well is dry, we have to dig deeper.

In her book *Passion and Purity*, Elisabeth Elliot comments about God's purposes in "unanswered prayer": "The deepest spiritual lessons are not learned by His letting us have our way in the end, but by His making us wait, bearing with us in love and patience until we are able to honestly pray what He taught His disciples to pray: Thy will be done."[1]

When we pray, God sometimes miraculously changes our circumstances, but more often, He changes us. He refocuses our attention on Him and His promises instead of our problems; He reminds us that He's God and we're not; and He gives us assurance that He'll accomplish His purposes, but not necessarily ours. Is that enough for us? Maybe, maybe not.

At different points and in different circumstances all of us come to a crisis of faith. Will we cling to God or drift away? Will we trust in His goodness when we don't see evidence of it? Will we wait on His answers when our pain screams for relief right now?

The temptation to be angry with God for not coming through isn't new to our circumstances. As we've seen, the Christians in Corinth were jealous of each other, fought and blamed, and they needed a strong hand to correct them. In Paul's first letter he set them straight about a lot of things. He gave them a stern warning coupled with tender assurance. Paul ran through a list of the ways God provided for Moses and the people of God in the wilderness, and he explained that many times they had turned their backs on God. Paul wrote, "So, if you think you are standing firm, be careful that you don't fall! No temptation has overtaken you except what is common to mankind. And God is faithful; he will not let you be tempted beyond what you can bear. But when you are tempted, he will also provide a way out so that you can endure it" (1 Cor. 10:12–13).

When we feel like giving up, God is there. When we believe all hope is lost, God has a plan. When we feel crushed under the weight of worries, God says, "Trust Me. I have a way forward."

## POUR OUT YOUR HEART

As we've seen, about half of the psalms describe elements of emotional distress, and their presence in God's Book—in fact, in God's songbook—tells us that it's more than OK to be honest with God about our anger and anxiety. The psalms are prayers as well as songs. David, Asaph, the sons of Korah, and other writers invite us to speak with raw truth as we address a good, wise, and powerful God. In an earlier chapter we saw the importance of feeling the full range of emotions; now we see the importance of expressing them in prayer.

In Psalm 62 David is again complaining that his enemies are about to get him. (This is a common theme in David's songs.) This time they are attempting a coup, and they're spreading lies to ruin his reputation. Have you ever been there? Many of us have experienced the pain of misunderstanding, and worse, the heartbreak of people lying to ruin us. I know I have. David complains:

> How long will you assault me? Would all of you throw me down—this leaning wall, this tottering fence? Surely they intend to topple me from my lofty place; they take delight in lies. With their mouths they bless, but in their hearts they curse.
>
> —Psalm 62:3–4

This is the crucial point: David finds peace and hope *before* the Lord changes his circumstances. In the middle of his pain, David's prayer revolutionizes his perspective:

> Yes, my soul, find rest in God; my hope comes from him. Truly he is my rock and my salvation; he is my fortress, I will not be shaken. My salvation and my honor depend on God; he is my mighty rock, my refuge.
>
> —Psalm 62:5–7

How did the change happen? Did David ignore the situation so he didn't have to think about it? Did he fill his mind with "happy talk" to convince himself that it wasn't as bad as it looked? Did he crater in despair because he had no hope at all? No, none of those. He went to God and poured out his heart in prayer. He held nothing back, and in the crucible of raw honesty, God met him. In the next verse, David's advice for others when they're distressed is to follow his example:

> Trust in him at all times, you people; pour out your
> hearts to him, for God is our refuge.
>
> —PSALM 62:8

A few of us trust God's mercy so much that we have no trouble coming to Him and pouring our hearts out, but most of us are hesitant. Maybe we didn't feel safe being completely honest with our parents, and we've transferred our reserve to our relationship with God. Or maybe we've believed the myth that "good Christians" are never angry or anxious, so we've convinced ourselves that the only emotions we can express to God are joy and gratitude. Or maybe we've never been in any relationship in which we felt safe enough to take our guard down. Whatever the reason for our reticence, we need to address it, correct it, and express our hearts to God.

The presence of the Book of Job, the "wintry" psalms, the despair of Paul, the depression of Elijah, and the heartache of Jesus reinforce to us that God isn't aloof, He doesn't demand only pleasant prayers, and we aren't alone. These passages shout that God is as merciful as He is powerful, as kind as He is wise.

## TEMPLATES

When we don't know how to pray, we can look to the Scriptures for help. God has graciously given us a lot of examples of heartfelt prayer. We can use these to guide us.

### The Psalms

We've seen how the Psalms are rich with honest expressions of emotions. The Psalms are also wonderful resources to guide our prayers. Sometimes when our hearts are full of God's goodness and greatness, we pray with David in Psalm 23.

> The LORD is my shepherd, I lack nothing. He makes me lie down in green pastures, he leads me beside quiet waters, he refreshes my soul. He guides me along the right paths for his name's sake.
>
> —PSALM 23:1–3

But shockingly, David's song just before this one is filled with heartache. He began with an expression of desolation that Jesus echoed on the cross.

> My God, my God, why have you forsaken me? Why are you so far from saving me, so far from my cries of anguish? My God, I cry out by day, but you do not answer, by night, but I find no rest.
>
> —PSALM 22:1–2

That was Francine's prayer, and it may be yours and mine from time to time. For most of the psalm David complains that his pain and his enemies are overwhelming him, but as he pours out his heart in anguish, God gives him renewed hope. The turning point is this request:

> But you, LORD, do not be far from me. You are my strength; come quickly to help me. Deliver me from the sword, my precious life from the power of the dogs. Rescue me from the mouth of the lions; save me from the horns of the wild oxen.
>
> —PSALM 22:19–21

David must have gotten some assurance that God would—somehow, someday—answer this prayer, because in the following verses he anticipates a time when he will praise God with all his heart.

> I will declare your name to my people; in the assembly
> I will praise you. You who fear the LORD, praise him!
> All you descendants of Jacob, honor him! Revere him,
> all you descendants of Israel! For he has not despised
> or scorned the suffering of the afflicted one; he has
> not hidden his face from him but has listened to his
> cry for help.
>
> —PSALM 22:22–24

David didn't get to the point of praise easily or quickly, but he got there eventually. It's often the same for us: as we wrestle with our discouragement and pour out our hearts to God, we'll gain His perspective, we'll sense His peace, and He'll renew our hope—sooner or later.

### The Lord's Prayer

In the Gospels we see Jesus praying early in the morning, all night, during the day, in the temple, in the synagogues, and on the mountainsides. His disciples were obviously impressed as they watched Him, so they asked, "Lord, teach us to pray." He gave them what we call the Lord's Prayer. The request for "daily bread" doesn't come first; in fact, it is only a small part of the prayer and follows many crucial reflections.

- What it means to call God "our Father"—we
  can call Him our Father only because Jesus paid

the price for us to be forgiven and we've been
adopted as God's beloved children;

- What it means to "hallow" the Father's name—all
of God's attributes (including His love, wisdom,
and power) are perfect and immeasurable;

- What it means to want God's kingdom to come—
His kingdom includes His reign later in perfect
glory and now through His people living out
God's kindness, righteousness, and justice; and

- What it means for His will to be done on earth as
it is in heaven—that we have ambidextrous faith,
trusting that God will use anything and everything for our good and His glory.

When our hearts are saturated with this perspective about
God and His purposes, we can then ask Him to provide our
daily bread, which I believe is much more than a loaf; it's a
sense of God's presence and power, opportunities to serve
Him, and the joy of watching Him change lives…as well as
meeting our needs for sustenance and shelter.

Many Protestants are wary of praying the Lord's Prayer
because we don't want to mouth it without meaning. However,
when we use each clause as a jumping-off point to think more
deeply and pray more fervently, it becomes a template that pro-
pels our prayers to new places.

### Paul's prayers

Over the years I've gotten a lot out of reflecting on Paul's
prayers in his letters to the churches. They show me how he

prayed, what was on his heart, and how he tapped into God's truth to strengthen his faith. His prayer in the opening chapter of the letter to the Ephesians is just what I need when I feel anxious. God brought this letter to my attention in my undergraduate studies in Greek exegesis.

Paul begins with gratitude for the believers, and he begins his request by asking for the same thing in two different ways: "I keep asking that the God of our Lord Jesus Christ, the glorious Father, may give you the Spirit of wisdom and revelation, so that you may know him better" (Eph. 1:17). How does God give us "the Spirit of wisdom and revelation"? By supernaturally "enlightening" the eyes of our hearts. The heart of his prayer focuses on three requests: for hope, riches, and power. Let's look at those.

Paul asks God to give the Ephesians spiritual perception to "know the hope to which [God] has called you" (v. 18). We often think of our hope as the promise of heaven. It's that, but it's much more. Our "calling" isn't only heaven, and it's not a role in the church. God calls us to be His children, to know Him, to love Him, and to follow Him. The people in the church in Ephesus (and us, too) didn't have to wonder what Paul meant because he spent the first part of this chapter describing our calling. Because God's grace is poured out on us through Christ, we've been chosen, adopted, forgiven, and sealed by the Holy Spirit as God's own (vv. 3–14). So, in the prayer, Paul asks God to make our hope in this calling so real that we know it experientially—with heart knowledge, not just head knowledge—so that we're overcome with wonder that the Creator has made us His own.

The second petition is for riches, but Paul isn't talking about money or possessions. He asks God to open the eyes of their hearts to know "the riches of his glorious inheritance in his holy people" (v. 18). Scholars aren't sure if Paul means that we're rich because we have God or that God considers Himself to be rich because He has us. It appears that both are true. Certainly we're fabulously rich because we're the recipients of God's great grace, but both Exodus 19:5 and 1 Peter 2:9 refer to us as "God's special possession." As the Exodus passage is translated, the word means "treasure." Get this: God considers you and me to be His treasure! Paul is praying that this truth will penetrate our hearts, shatter our despair, and renew our joy.

The third request is that we would know "his incomparably great power for us who believe" (v. 19). But that's not enough for Paul! He describes this power as "the same as the mighty strength he exerted when he raised Christ from the dead and seated him at his right hand in the heavenly realms" (vv. 19–20). Paul goes on to say that Jesus has authority over every power, seen and unseen, and is the head of the church, His body. We usually think of God's power in miraculous healings, creation, and other dramatic events, but we get a glimpse of the purpose of this power in Paul's prayer in the opening chapter of Colossians. There he prays that the Christians will be "strengthened with all power according to his glorious might so that you may have great endurance and patience" (Col. 1:11). In other words, at least one of the reasons we need the supernatural power of the Holy Spirit is for endurance and patience. Isn't that exactly what we need when we're fearful, anxious, and discouraged? Strength in times of trial doesn't just magically appear; it's the result of the Spirit of God giving us perspective, renewing our hope, and assuring us that He will do what only He can do.

I pray the prayer in the first chapter of Ephesians for myself, my family, my friends, my colleagues, my pastor, and for our nation. It's a wonderful jumping-off point for me because each of the three parts of the petition—hope, riches, and power—changes my perspective, rivets my hope on God, and inspires me to trust God for more.

## MORE THAN EVER

Troubled times are watersheds for our spiritual lives. Heartache either drives us closer to God or further from Him—and if we're honest, many of us would say that our biggest problems first were barriers in our connection with God, but they became paths of growth. When life makes no sense, prayer becomes a lifeline—not to magically make everything all better all at once, but to take us deeper into the heart of God. There we find Him to be good and great. If He were only good, we might have pleasant feelings about Him, but we wouldn't trust Him to do a powerful work at the depths of our hearts. And if we only see Him as great, we might think of Him as a mighty king, but one who isn't necessarily concerned about us. No, our God is infinitely good *and* infinitely great. We can come to Him, pour out our hearts, ask Him for anything, and rest in the fact that He will accomplish His purposes. No wonder Psalm 46:1 reminds us that God is our refuge and strength and a very present help during our time of trouble. Hold on to Him and that promise.

Think about it:

1. What percentage of your prayers are asking God to change your circumstances, and what percentage are requests for Him to change you? What does this tell you about your prayers?

2. When we're distressed, we often think we're at the end of our ropes. How do you respond to God's comment that He will never give us more than we can handle (1 Cor. 10:13)?

3. Are you at all resistant to pour your heart out to God? Explain your answer.

4. Which of the templates for prayer do you want to use? How will it (they) help you refocus your prayers, your expectations, and your hopes?

5. Why is it important to see God as both infinitely good and infinitely great?

# Chapter 8

# DO IT

*A Christian's freedom from anxiety is not due to some guaranteed freedom from trouble, but to the folly of worry...and especially to the confidence that God is our Father, that even permitted suffering is within the orbit of His care.*

—JOHN STOTT, *THE MESSAGE OF THE SERMON ON THE MOUNT*

FOR ALMOST THE entire hour of her appointment Marsha talked about the stress she was experiencing. She described her troubled marriage, the strained relationships with her sons, her husband's terrible financial decisions and the weight of debt they carried, how her best friends had abandoned her, and that she was terrified someone close to her would get COVID-19. I listened—and I continued to listen. It was obvious that she really needed to feel heard and understood. That was important. Near the end, I validated her feelings and perceptions: "Marsha, no wonder you feel so much stress. Troubles have been coming at you from all directions." She nodded. Then I asked, "Tell me, how are you managing your anxiety?"

She responded like I'd asked her if she knew any Martians. I tried again. "There are some simple things people can do to lower their level of stress. Are you using any of them?"

Marsha frowned and said, "I didn't think it was a good idea for me to bury all my feelings." She still didn't understand my question.

"No, of course not. But are you getting regular exercise? Are you doing some things you enjoy? Do you have a plan to deal with the financial pressures? Things like that."

Marsha seemed perplexed. "I…I'm not doing any of those things. I spend all my time worrying."

Marsha isn't alone in this response to stress. Many of us fail to take action. We're very aggressive in our worrying, but we're passive in managing our stress. We can do better. As anxieties multiply in the wake of the first wave of the pandemic and hot spots continue to arise, we must do better if we're going to be sane and purposeful.

In this chapter I want to be very prescriptive. We'll look at a number of very practical steps you can take to reduce your level of anxiety.

## A COUNSELOR'S EYES AND EARS

We won't be able to take effective action if we haven't identified the problem. You can't treat what you don't see. As we've seen in the previous chapters, being honest about our difficult situations and the emotions that accompany them is the trigger to our managing and reducing levels of stress. How many of these effects are true for you, and to what level of severity?

___ Your mind is consumed with the "dark side" of what might happen.

___ Your emotions are on edge.

___ You've become stir-crazy, or you only feel safe at home—or both.

___ You can't seem to find words to describe how you feel and what you want to do.

___ You're exhausted from the constant worry.

___ You forget important tasks at home and at work, tasks you routinely performed before.

___ You feel muscle tension, you have frequent headaches, or you have digestive problems.

___ You don't laugh much, and when you do, it's at the wrong things.

___ You cry much more than normal, or you never cry.

___ You find fault with everybody and everything.

___ You can't seem to find any relief from the burden of your worries.

___ You're having panic attacks.

The stresses throughout our nation and the world have multiplied with the pandemic. We already had enough trouble without it, but now sickness, death, isolation, unemployment, losses in retirement funds, mounting bills, kids going stir-crazy, and disruption in the delivery of necessities have given us plenty of reasons to feel the burdens of painful certainties and fearful uncertainties. We need a plan. We need to do the things we've always known to do, but now we need them more than ever.

As we take steps to manage our stress, there are some things most of us can do, and there are things some of us need to do.

## FOR MOST OF US

"When I worry, my brain goes to mush." William almost laughed when he said this to me…almost. He was expressing a common problem for people who are under inordinate pressure: instead of thinking more clearly, we're often more confused. In these times we need clearly defined, attainable goals and steps to help us move forward. It's important to start with one or two and see success than to try a dozen and become even more discouraged. I'll offer a number of suggestions, but please, start small and build from there.

### 1. Connect.

In normal times, stress often causes people to withdraw from others. Having regular conversations is just too hard, so it's easier to avoid them. But now all of us have experienced "social distancing" for weeks or months, and some of us are in at-risk communities and need to continue to self-isolate to some extent. But God has made us social creatures—we need each other like we need air and water.

I've been very encouraged to see reports of families and friends finding creative ways to connect online using video platforms, and neighbors have come out of their houses to stand on opposite sides of the street to see how the others are coping. This, I'm convinced, is the most important step for us.

You may feel the urge to isolate, but fight it. You may not be able to have the same kind of contact that you did before and will, we trust, have again, so creativity and tenacity are essential.

Whatever you do, stay connected. Make the call, send the text, see the faces and hear the voices on video calls, and talk to neighbors. You need it, they need it, we all need it.

## 2. Deepen the connections.

I've talked to parents of young children who used the time during lockdowns to read to their kids far more than they used to. Some have time to play games, take walks, and show their children the wonders of nature. Couples haven't been as rushed to get to the office or go to meetings, and they've found more time to talk about what's important, our desire to have heart connections that were being crowded out by their busy schedules.

It's certainly tempting to binge-watch shows on Amazon or Netflix, but it's wise to set some limits so the habit of watching television doesn't prevent meaningful conversations.

I've also heard from people who said they've cooked more than ever before. They may still get takeout from time to time, but many are calling their mothers or grandmothers to talk about recipes or their fathers and grandfathers to ask how to smoke the world's best ribs.

At this point most of us don't see as many people as we did before the coronavirus, but we can have deeper, richer, more meaningful connections with the ones who are still in our orbit.

### 3. Find something to make you smile and laugh.

Yes, things are serious. Yes, people are sick and dying, the economy has taken a hit, and we're all trying to find ways to cope with the stress. It's easy to be overwhelmed with worry, so we need even more to find things that amuse us, stimulate our creativity, and make us say, "Wow!"

We need to be students of the people around us. What do they enjoy? What makes them laugh until they're about to throw up? What makes them so excited that they can't wait to tell you about it? If we can identify those things, we can create moments with them that thrill them…which in turn brings us joy.

The list of activities and games is endless. We might try magic tricks or juggling, new recipes, charades, board games, a game of catch, fishing, dodgeball, or acting out a drama somebody has just written.

We need to laugh, we need to have a sense of wonder, we need thrills. And we need these especially when life is hard.

### 4. Establish healthy rhythms.

When we're at home all the time because of lockdowns (complete or partial), we can lose the habits that made us successful and happy. We may sleep longer, eat more, and lounge more than before, or we may sleep and eat too little and be distracted from the things that matter. When we're under stress, we need good, workable rhythms more than ever. Set your alarm for the morning, buy only healthy foods (with maybe a few indulgences to keep life interesting), and create a schedule that works for you and those in your home.

As you consider the rhythms, you'll set priorities. My wife,

Julie, is really strong here. These may have shifted in the past few months—it seems everything has shifted! Take time to think through what's most important, what's fairly important, and what's completely negotiable or expendable. As they say, "Major on the majors" and get to the rest when and if you can.

### 5. Make a financial plan.

Before the pandemic many of us were living paycheck to paycheck and spending every dime we earned. We ignored advice to have several months of money in a "rainy day fund," and now it's too late to start one. Debts are rising, income has diminished, and we feel the squeeze. This may be just the wake-up call we need to force us to make better decisions about money. We may have assumed we didn't need a budget, but we certainly need one now. We may have spent money on anything that interested us, but no longer.

One of the biggest burdens of debt is not knowing how to get out of it. Many people give up and don't make the changes they could make to get out of debt and have a firm financial footing. This is the time. Go online, read a book, or talk to someone who has good answers, and create a plan that works for you and your family. Implementing the strategy may be difficult, but it won't be as stressful as not having a plan.

### 6. Keep a journal.

When we're anxious, our minds often race from one worry to another and back again, making loops that make us even more frantic and hopeless. Keeping a journal encourages clear thinking and good planning. You don't have to be Shakespeare to benefit. No one else needs to read what you write, so let it be just for you.

I encourage you to begin each day's entry with thanksgiving. Reflect on the good things God has given you before you pour your heart out with concerns. It's also wise to let your writing shape your actions. Gradually or suddenly your reflections clarify your direction and give you specific steps to take.

Some people buy a book with blank pages so they have an investment in journaling. Whether you buy one of these, you use notebook paper, or you type on your computer, dive in and let the process shape your thoughts, galvanize your emotions, and prod you to action.

### 7. Let it go.

When we're on edge, people get on our nerves. Words or actions that didn't matter to us before now get under our skin. We're more easily annoyed, offended, and royally hacked off! And we're probably getting on others' nerves too! Times of increased stress are opportunities to practice the fine art of forgiving and apologizing—to let it go.

Forgiveness doesn't come naturally, but give it a try. When we're hurt, we want to lash back or run and hide. But as Christians we have a bottomless well of grace that God has given us in Christ. Paul explained to the believers in Ephesus: "Get rid of all bitterness, rage and anger, brawling and slander, along with every form of malice. Be kind and compassionate to one another, forgiving each other, just as in Christ God forgave you. Follow God's example, therefore, as dearly loved children and walk in the way of love, just as Christ loved us and gave himself up for us as a fragrant offering and sacrifice to God" (Eph. 4:31–5:2).

We can be kind and compassionate because God has been so kind and compassionate with us. And we can forgive because God has poured out His forgiveness on us through Christ's sacrifice. We can love because we're the recipients of God's amazing love. When we have a hard time forgiving, we look at Jesus and remember what He did for us. Still, forgiveness isn't easy. In *The Reason for God* author and pastor Tim Keller explains this.

> Forgiveness means refusing to make them pay for what they did. However, to refrain from lashing out at someone when you want to do so with all your being is *agony*. It is a form of suffering. You not only suffer the original loss of happiness, reputation, and opportunity, but now you forgo the consolation of inflicting the same on them. You are absorbing the debt, taking the cost of it completely on yourself instead of taking it out of the other person. It hurts terribly. Many people would say it feels like a kind of death. Yes, but it is a death that leads to resurrection instead of the lifelong living death of bitterness and cynicism.[1]

To some extent forgiveness always involves a measure of grief because we're forgiving someone for taking something from us—a possession, perhaps, but more likely happiness, security, or our good name. So we probably won't have pleasant, happy feelings when we choose to forgive; we'll have a realization of the loss. But the bitterness and self-pity will slowly dissolve.

But the shoe is on the other foot just as often. We've been annoying, we've been petty, we've blamed, and we've harmed. We need to apologize and ask for forgiveness. The person may not instantly hug us and say everything is fine, because he or she now needs to grieve as well as forgive.

Forgiveness is a rare thing, but when it happens, it's beautiful. It is the essence of the Christian faith, and it's the foundation of strong relationships. I'd say that people who never have to forgive or be forgiven are either living alone on another planet or have very superficial relationships. It's a skill and a habit all of us need to acquire...especially during hard times when emotions are raw and nerves are frayed.

### 8. Communicate with children in age-appropriate ways.

In the past decade or so our culture has experienced a major shift in parenting. Years ago we required good performance to earn As in school, awards in sports, and praise at home, but no longer. The goal of parenting has changed: We used to do whatever it takes to prepare our children to be mature, responsible adults, which included letting them suffer the consequences of poor choices. But today the goal of many parents is to protect their kids from any unpleasantness at all. Our schools give higher grades for the same performance as before, our kids' athletic teams give everyone a "participant's trophy," and many of us can't stand it if our kids are the least bit unhappy—about anything.

The shift is a problem in the best of times, but it's destructive during the anxiety of any calamity, including the pandemic.

The urge to shield our kids keeps them from processing their fear and learning lessons that can only be acquired during hardships.

When we don't talk to our children about what's going on or tell them about our fears, we miss a golden opportunity to connect with them and impart God's wisdom. The fact is that they sense our anxiety. It's written on our faces and is heard in our voices—and they absorb the fear in the home's atmosphere just like they absorb oxygen from the air they breathe. Healthy parents are attuned to those needs.

Of course, we need to communicate with our kids in age-appropriate ways. The younger ones need more reassurance that they're loved and safe. Older children, especially teenagers and young adults, need more honesty from us. We can tell them we're worried and afraid. And we can invite them to be honest about their painful emotions—without discounting them or trying to fix them. Our gifts to them are a patient, listening ear; emotional authenticity; and genuine hope. That will go a lot further in helping them wrestle with the crisis than simplistic answers, emotional cover-ups, and empty platitudes neither they nor we believe.

### 9. Avoid the misuse of substances.

When we're stressed, we turn to all kinds of things to soothe our fragmented souls. If we used alcohol in moderation before, we're now tempted to drink too much. If we smoked or vaped, we use nicotine in increasing measures. And if we enjoyed caffeine before, we may drink too many cups of coffee or too many soft drinks—yikes! That's getting too close to home!

In the United States during the middle of the first wave of

the pandemic, alcohol sales rose 55 percent, and online sales were up a staggering 243 percent.[2] Much of that, it's assumed, happened as people stocked up as stay-at-home orders were enacted.

The misuse and abuse of substances is a big problem today because people have plenty of reasons to self-medicate and either self-soothe or add some artificial energy to their exhausted bodies. Don't give in to the temptation.

## 10. Worship.

I'm not talking about going to church. By the time you're reading this, I hope our churches are open again, but new hot spots of the virus may limit large group gatherings for a while in certain communities. Whatever the circumstances, we need to fill our hearts with the wonder, majesty, and kindness of God. That's what I mean by worship. We certainly need to connect with Him in our private devotional times, but families can pray together and talk about passages of Scripture, and small groups can join on video platforms to study, pray, and encourage one another.

Worship isn't an ancillary activity. Anxiety may indicate many things, but it certainly means that our troubles threaten to overwhelm our sense of God's greatness and grace. I'm not suggesting we engage in superficial worship—far from it. Go back to the chapters in this book that encourage you to feel deeply, think clearly, and pray expectantly. That's what makes worship a powerful activity that transforms us from the inside out.

As I mentioned, it's not wise to try to implement too much too soon. Take a bite of one or two, chew on them until they become part of your routine and you see a difference in your outlook, and then bite on a couple more. Success breeds success, and you'll make glorious progress.

However, some of us need much more help.

## FOR SOME OF US

In some households during the pandemic, people aren't just annoyed with each other; they're harming each other. In an article about the rise in domestic abuse, Amanda Taub observes:

> Add another public health crisis to the toll of the new coronavirus: Mounting data suggests that domestic abuse is acting like an opportunistic infection, flourishing in the conditions created by the pandemic....Domestic violence goes up whenever families spend more time together, such as the Christmas and summer vacations....Now, with families in lockdown worldwide, hotlines are lighting up with abuse reports, leaving governments trying to address a crisis that experts say they should have seen coming.[3]

During the lockdown the incidences of domestic abuse rose 25 percent in countries throughout the world.[4] Along with the increased sale of alcohol, gun sales are the highest ever recorded since the national instant check system for buyers began in 1998.[5] Unemployment and the stay-at-home orders are keeping couples at home, and they face the combined pressure of mounting debt, the frustration of delays, and the demands of children. Those who were already prone to violence now have very little margin, and those who were protected by distance at work are vulnerable.

Therapist Jason Whiting reports a session with a woman named Sheila, whose husband, Gus, lost his job in the coronavirus lockdown. She explained that Gus had been sleeping during the day and watching violent videos at night. When they were both awake at the same time, "he was demanding, insisting that she feed him or run to the liquor store. After several days of this, she refused. He then took her car keys, yelled at her, and accused her of 'nagging' and 'provoking' him.... He was making suicidal threats and becoming physical, pushing Sheila away when she wanted to talk, and holding her down when she tried to leave." When the therapist asked if she feels safe, Sheila replied, "I don't think he would really hurt me, but I have never seen him this out of control."[6]

If you or someone you love is a victim or a perpetrator of domestic violence, take action. If you wait, something much worse might happen. Call a women's shelter, the police, your pastor, or a counselor. You can expect the perpetrator to deny the charge, and many if not most of the victims are too scared of reprisals to be honest. Still, make the call.

For some the effects of anxiety are beyond normal. They suffer from anxiety disorders or panic attacks. The disorder is diagnosed when worry is overwhelming and interferes with relationships and the functions of daily life. Symptoms vary, but they often include hypervigilance (always watching for signs of danger), irritability, feelings of gloom and dread, having your mind go blank, or having intrusive thoughts you can't control. The physiological symptoms that are common in stress—muscle tension, headaches, insomnia, heart pounding, and digestive problems—are amplified in an anxiety disorder.

Panic attacks are sudden episodes of intense fear, usually appearing without warning, but also associated with triggers like feeling claustrophobic in an MRI, getting stuck in an elevator, hearing unidentified sounds at night, or being tasked with giving a speech. In addition to the sudden, overwhelming fear, panic attacks may include shortness of breath, heart palpitations, hot flashes or chills, shaking, nausea, or feeling detached from reality.

The recommendations I've given in this chapter can help people who struggle with the more severe forms of anxiety, but in addition I strongly recommend professional help. A therapist can help people uncover the source of the anxiety, provide tools to control it, and perhaps work with a physician to prescribe appropriate medications.

Anxiety disorders and panic attacks aren't signs of moral flaws or spiritual weakness. They often have a genetic or biological component, and they have connections with emotional wounds that have never healed. Occasionally medical conditions such as thyroid problems or asthma can contribute to anxiety disorders and panic attacks, and sometimes prescriptions for other health concerns can increase levels of anxiety.

If these descriptions fit you, see a physician as well as a therapist, and get the help you need to manage stress and lower your level of worry.

## NEVER ALONE, NEVER HELPLESS

After Joanne explained that she has fought for years to over-come her fears, she said with a tear in her eye, "I've been this way all my life. I don't guess it'll ever be any different." I assured her that hope isn't lost. We're never alone because we have the Spirit of God living inside us, and we're never help-less because God will help us climb out of the hole that we're in. Relief may not come quickly, but it will come. I love David's blend of honesty and hope in this psalm:

> I waited patiently for the LORD; he turned to me and heard my cry. He lifted me out of the slimy pit, out of the mud and mire; he set my feet on a rock and gave me a firm place to stand. He put a new song in my mouth, a hymn of praise to our God. Many will see and fear the LORD and put their trust in him.
>
> —PSALM 40:1–3

When we've suffered from stress for a long time and don't see light at the end of the tunnel, it's easy to think it will always be like this. Actually that's true—unless we think clearly to identify the steps we need to take and find the courage to take the first one. Trust Him, climb out of the pit, and take steps toward a healthier, happier, more purposeful life.

Think about it:

1. Look back at the list of the effects of stress in the beginning of this chapter, and then rate your experience of each one from 0 (not in the least) to 10 (all day every day).

Which three were your highest scores?

Describe how these have affected your mood, your relationships, and your hope for the future.

2. In the section called "For Most of Us," what is the one thing (or at most, what are the two things) you want to incorporate into your life first?

   Why did you pick this (or these)?
   What's your plan?
   What difference will it (or they) make?

3. Were you surprised that I included worship as an action point to manage anxiety? Explain your answer.

4. Are you or someone you love in an abusive relationship? What steps can you take for protection?

5. How can you support people who are overwhelmed with an anxiety disorder or suffer from panic attacks?

*Chapter 9*

# LESSONS LEARNED

*A God wise enough to create me and the world I
live in is wise enough to watch out for me.*

—PHILIP YANCEY, *WHERE IS GOD WHEN IT HURTS?*

A QUICK LOOK AT Amazon brings up a surprising number of books with the titles *Don't Waste Your Pain* and *Don't Waste Your Sorrows*. The titles reflect one of the biggest challenges we'll ever face, and it's very good advice. Calamity reinforces calamity if we fail to learn the lessons God wants to teach us from sudden heartaches and prolonged strains. In this final chapter I want to identify at least some of the most important lessons we can learn.

## GOD'S AGENDA IS ALWAYS BIGGER

If we gain even a moderate amount of self-awareness during stressful seasons in our lives, we realize that our goals—our real goals—are always much smaller than God's...and often in opposition to His. Our first realization of this truth may startle us, but it shouldn't surprise us much after that. With a new level of humility we admit we aren't in control, we don't know what's best, and we can't guarantee outcomes.

Some scholars believe the prophet Isaiah was a proud young man, but when God appeared in the temple in fire and glory (in Isaiah 6), Isaiah's pride was crushed under a new reality of his smallness. He became God's servant, even though he protested that no one would listen to him. Much later in the book he wrote for us, Isaiah gives us a glimpse of the lesson he learned as he quotes God.

> "For my thoughts are not your thoughts, neither are your ways my ways," declares the LORD. "As the heavens are higher than the earth, so are my ways higher than your ways and my thoughts than your thoughts. As the rain and the snow come down from heaven, and do not return to it without watering the earth and making it bud and flourish, so that it yields seed for the sower and bread for the eater, so is my word that goes out from my mouth: It will not return to me empty, but will accomplish what I desire and achieve the purpose for which I sent it."
>
> —ISAIAH 55:8–11

We may think we know better than God how life ought to go, but our thoughts only produce worry and resentment when things don't work out like we plan. God's agenda is always far bigger, far more complicated, and far better than we can imagine. Our assumptions of omniscience get me (and the rest of us) into big trouble!

When we aren't humbled by God's infinite wisdom and purposes, we often ask the wrong questions. At one point Jesus and His disciples saw a man who had been blind from birth. The disciples were sure the condition had one of two possible causes. John takes us to the scene.

His disciples asked him, "Rabbi, who sinned, this man or his parents, that he was born blind?"

"Neither this man nor his parents sinned," said Jesus, "but this happened so that the works of God might be displayed in him. As long as it is day, we must do the works of him who sent me. Night is coming, when no one can work. While I am in the world, I am the light of the world."

—JOHN 9:2–5

The disciples couldn't see any deeper or higher purpose for the man's blindness. They only wanted to pin the blame on somebody. Jesus assured them that this man's problem—and every person's problem—is part of a far bigger story of redemption. Jesus made mud from the most common elements of dirt and spit, and He did the incredible, the awe inspiring, the miraculous. He opened the man's eyes so he could see.

A measure of concern and anxiety is good—they're the right response to heartache and loss. But when we think we know what God should do, and we insist on Him doing it, we slide into corrosive worry, rising anxiety, and hopelessness. The lesson God wants to teach us is that even when we don't have a clue, He knows exactly what He's doing, so we can trust Him. Is it hard to do? Yes.

## SET PRIORITIES

When our minds are scattered and our hearts are burdened, we need to examine our priorities and recalibrate them. We're familiar with the time Jesus and His followers went to Bethany for lunch with His friends Mary and Martha. As Jesus sat in the living room talking about things that matter, Martha was frantically preparing lunch. When she finally had a conversation with Jesus, it wasn't about the kingdom! She complained, blaming Him and her sister: "Lord, don't you care that my sister has left me to do the work by myself? Tell her to help me!" (Luke 10:40).

I can almost see the smile on Jesus' face as He answered her. "Martha, Martha…you are worried and upset about many things, but few things are needed—or indeed only one. Mary has chosen what is better, and it will not be taken away from her" (Luke 10:41–42).

Lockdowns, social distancing, unemployment, piles of debt, sickness, and death have revealed what's really important to us. When times were better (if not great), many of us were focused on responses to our social media posts, the next promotion at work, a great vacation, clothes, our bank accounts, and having fun. When those things were taken away, or at least threatened, how did we respond? Did we hide behind the myths we examined earlier in the book? Did we complain incessantly? Or did we take the opportunity to recalibrate our hearts and our priorities? It's still not too late.

We may have avoided deep reflection and the challenge of repentance before, but now we realize that we aren't going to make it if we can't get God's perspective on what's happening. And it doesn't take much to realize that our response has been something less than stellar! Repentance is agreeing with God that we've been off base, maybe blown it, that He has already forgiven us through Christ's sacrifice, and that His path is preferable to the one we've charted for ourselves. Humble people have learned the art and skill of repenting. If you haven't learned it, now's the time.

## Honesty and Growth

We won't grow if we're not honest about our need to grow. We won't get stronger and wiser until we admit we're weak and foolish apart from God's intervention. We don't need Him less; we need Him more. As we've seen, some of us are overwhelmed with our emotions, and they dominate our thoughts, actions, and relationships. But others have put clamps on their hearts so they don't feel the sadness, fear, resentment, and self-pity. Whether we admit it or not, those emotions are in all of us to one degree or another.

We saw that the Book of Psalms is our example of being raw in our relationship with God. The writers poured out their hearts, and God met them where they were. He didn't demand that they get their acts together before He assured them of His love and plans. When they were at their worst, He was at His best to comfort, guide, and reassure them.

The Scriptures, and especially the Psalms, are an amazing repository of brutal honesty. In his commentary on one of them Derek Kidner comments, "The very presence of such prayers in Scripture is a witness to his understanding. He knows how men speak when they are desperate."[1]

Are you desperate? God is waiting for you to come to Him and follow the lead of the psalmists: tell God exactly what you think and how you feel, and let Him meet you there. This process will feel very uncomfortable—and wrong—to many of us, but it's essential if we want to tap into God's vast treasure of grace, mercy, wisdom, and strength.

## NOT THE SAME

Stress comes in many forms and in a range of degrees. Some of us have been devastated by the death of someone we love because of the virus, many have lost their jobs and incomes, and all of us have experienced no small measure of inconvenience. Some communities, like New York, have seen far more disease and death than other parts of the country, but most of us have missed the ravages of COVID-19.

Similarly, we have different personalities, different life experiences, and different coping skills. Some feel more deeply than others, and some are more logical—and they're often married to each other!

The point is that we make a mistake when we assume people should handle stress the way we do. There are no "shoulds" in this. We need to give people, including our children, room to wrestle with their emotions and assumptions however they need to. Some of us make quick decisions and draw instant conclusions, but most people need longer to process their responses. We need to give them plenty of time.

## DEVELOP A NEW SKILL: LISTEN

When we're stressed, it seems like our IQ goes down because we're distracted and make dumb decisions, our patience evaporates under the incessant demands, and our relational talents are eroded because we're preoccupied with our problems. But the people around us are going through the same struggles, and they need us.

I'll be honest: When I'm under the gun, my adrenaline kicks in like a jet engine, and I frantically run around trying to fix things. Many things get left behind (like sanity), and the one that's most damaging is my willingness to listen. It sounds simple, doesn't it: just listen to people. But for many of us, it's the hardest thing to do. We're already swamped by our enormous difficulties, and we sure don't want to hear about anyone else's!

Years ago Pastor B. B. Warfield studied the life of Jesus, particularly passages about His emotions. He made a surprising discovery: the four Gospel writers described Jesus' compassion more than any other emotion. They said he often felt an "internal movement of pity," which prompted "an external act of beneficence."[2] The writers say that He was "moved with compassion," which is a translation of the Greek word that literally means He was "shaken in His bowels." Have you ever felt another person's pain so deeply that your insides shook? That's how Jesus responded to people in need…and that's how He still responds when we're in need. When we say we're followers of Christ, it means we take on His purpose and His heart for people. And when we're moved with compassion for our spouses, our kids, our parents, our neighbors, our friends, and others in our world, we'll take time to listen to them.

I know that I'm not listening when I'm thinking about the next thing I need to do or about how to answer so the conversation will be over as soon as possible. I know I'm not listening when I don't give eye contact, and when I interrupt to give my pearls of wisdom.

How do I know—and how does the other person know—I'm really listening? It's when I ask follow-up questions. Second and third questions invite the person to share more deeply and specifically. She knows I'm connecting. When I'm really clued in, I wait until the person has finished a thought, and then I say, "Here's what I hear you saying…" and I repeat it in my own words. This either gives tremendous validation to her, or she can say, "No, that's not quite it. Let me try again." And after the next attempt I say, "OK, I think I've got it. I think you're telling me…"

In times of crisis we're listening to people share their sorrows and heartaches, their confusion and bitterness, and their compulsion to blame somebody. These aren't pleasant conversations, but they're an essential part of the healing process for them…and maybe for us. When people begin to open up, don't shut them down. Take a deep breath, think about the compassion of Jesus, look the person in the eye, and really listen. It will do both of you a lot of good.

We can pay attention to the hurts and worries of others because Jesus pays attention to ours. Like all spiritual truth, we can't share what we don't possess, but we do possess the wealth of spiritual love and power. In other words, we love others out of the deep love we've experienced from God, we forgive because God has freely and completely forgiven us, and we accept people who are different from us because we were as different from Jesus as dark from light, yet He accepted us as His own. The willingness to listen is just the expression of a heart that has been melted and molded by the grace of God.

## The Deep Well

You and I have resources that many others don't have: the wisdom of the Word of God, the power of the Spirit of God, and the comfort of the people of God. However, under stress it's easy to see ourselves as desperately needy instead of being fabulously rich in God's blessings.

When we're convinced that we have those resources, we have more peace in our minds and hope in our hearts. We're more resilient, more honest, kinder, gentler, and stronger. We no longer need to play like we're someone we're not. At one point Paul thought he was beyond hope. He had endured physical suffering, betrayal by believers, attacks from outsiders, and the torment of the enemy. He prayed that God would rescue him, but He didn't answer the way Paul expected. In his second letter to the Corinthians he tells us how God spoke into his dilemma: "But he said to me, 'My grace is sufficient for you, for my power is made perfect in weakness.' Therefore I will boast all the more gladly about my weaknesses, so that Christ's power may rest on me. That is why, for Christ's sake, I delight in weaknesses, in insults, in hardships, in persecutions, in difficulties. For when I am weak, then I am strong" (2 Cor. 12:9–10).

Are you at the point of despair like Paul? If not, it's almost certain you will be at some point. God hasn't promised to protect us from trouble or to rescue us quickly, but He promises to give us grace and strength to endure it…and to learn the biggest lessons of life in the process.

Corrie ten Boom was a Dutch Christian. When the Nazis invaded, her family had a choice: to watch their Jewish neighbors be deported and murdered or risk their lives to help them. For two years she and her family protected Jewish families, but in February 1944 they were discovered in a Gestapo raid. Corrie, along with her sister Betsie, was sent to Ravensbruck, one of the concentration camps. In December of that year Betsie got sick and died. In the years after her release from the camp Corrie spoke often and eloquently about how dear she found Jesus in the horrors of the camp, and she often quoted Betsie's words of devotion and hope: "There is no pit so deep that God's love is not deeper still."[3]

That's the promise for us too.

## YOUR CHOICE

Suffering either pulverizes or strengthens. It's your choice. In the same letter to the Corinthians, Paul gave them a bracing perspective about facing hardships. Sufferings will come, he promises, but they give us unique opportunities to experience the power of God and be a beacon of light to those around us.

> But we have this treasure in jars of clay to show that this all-surpassing power is from God and not from us. We are hard pressed on every side, but not crushed; perplexed, but not in despair; persecuted, but not abandoned; struck down, but not destroyed. We always carry around in our body the death of

> Jesus, so that the life of Jesus may also be revealed in
> our body.
>
> —2 Corinthians 4:7–10

Does this inspire you or deflate you? Maybe both, to some extent. Paul's statement is the same as I've been trying to communicate throughout this book: at points in our lives heartaches are unavoidable, but God never abandons us, and He promises to use them to make us shine as lights to the people who are watching.

We've been through multiple shocks in the last year, and many experts are saying that things will never be quite the same. That was certainly true for Corrie and her family, but they found the courage to care, the courage to love, and the courage to hope. That's what Jesus is asking of you and me.

Pastor Rick Warren has enjoyed the phenomenal growth of his church, and he has suffered the devastating death of his son by suicide. He has earned the right to tell us something about the experience of pain: "When you shine the light of God's love through your circumstances, he can turn your pain into a beautiful picture. He develops your character through it. He makes you stronger. Most importantly, he uses your pain."[4]

Do you believe that? Are you convinced that God is using the trouble in our nation and your family to do something wonderful in you and through you?

Believe it. Hold on to it. Claim it. Do it. Why? Because it's true. Let me close with the prayer from Numbers 6:24–26: "The Lord bless you and keep you; the Lord make his face shine on you...and give you peace." A peace for your mind and hope for your heart.

Think about it:

1. What are some ways it helps to know that God's agenda is always bigger and better than ours?

2. How does stress reveal our true priorities?
    Do any of yours need to change? Explain your answer.

3. Why is it so hard to listen when we're under the gun?

4. How can you tell if someone is really listening to you?

5. Are you drawing from the deep well of the resources God has provided for you?
    How can you tell?
    How can you draw from them even more?

6. What's the most important lesson you've learned from this book?

# ABOUT THE AUTHOR

Tim Clinton, EdD, LPC, LMFT, is the president of the American Association of Christian Counselors (AACC), the largest and most diverse Christian counseling association in the world. Dr. Clinton also serves as the executive director of the James Dobson Family Institute and cohost of *Dr. James Dobson's Family Talk*, heard on nearly thirteen hundred radio outlets daily. Licensed as a professional counselor and a marriage and family therapist, Dr. Clinton is recognized as a world leader in mental health and relationship issues and has authored or edited nearly thirty books. He and his wife, Julie, have two children, Megan and Zach, and a granddaughter, Olivia.

# ABOUT THE AACC

THE AMERICAN ASSOCIATION of Christian Counselors (AACC) is the world's largest and most diverse Christian mental health organization, serving professional counselors, pastors, and lay leaders committed to biblical integrity and clinical excellence.

The AACC exists to bring honor to Jesus Christ; to encourage and promote excellence in counseling worldwide; to disseminate information, educational resources, and counseling aids; to inspire the highest level of counselor training; and to contribute to the strengthening of families.

Membership is available to mental health professionals, religious leaders, coaches, lay counselors, and others interested in Christian counseling but who have little to no professional training. AACC members enjoy numerous benefits and receive several publications, including the award-winning *Christian Counseling Today* magazine.

# NOTES

## CHAPTER 1

1. David Brooks, "The Pandemic of Fear and Agony," *New York Times*, April 9, 2020, https://www. nytimes.com/2020/04/09/opinion/covid-anxiety. html?campaignId=7JFJX.

2. David Brooks, "I Feel Like I'm Finally Cracking and I Don't Even Know Why," *New York Times*, April 9, 2020, https://www.nytimes.com/2020/04/09/opinion/mental-health-isolation-coronavirus.html.

3. Brooks, "The Pandemic of Fear and Agony"; Brooks, "I Feel Like I'm Finally Cracking and I Don't Even Know Why."

4. Gypsyamber D'Souza and David Dowdy, "What Is Herd Immunity and How Can We Achieve It With COVID-19?," Johns Hopkins Bloomberg School of Public Health, April 10, 2020, https://www.jhsph.edu/covid-19/articles/achieving-herd-immunity-with-covid19.html.

5. Jason Bisnoff, "Coronavirus Anxiety Hits Wealthy Investors Who Remain Pessimistic About Stocks and US Economy," *Forbes*, March 30, 2020, https://www. forbes.com/sites/jasonbisnoff/2020/03/30/coronavirus-anxiety-hits-wealthy-investors-who-remain-pessimistic-about-stocks-and-us-economy/#6d44ac9f4ca5; Erin Duffin, "US—Real GDP Growth by Year 1990–2019," Statista, February 3, 2020, https://www.statista.com/statistics/188165/annual-gdp-growth-of-the-united-states-since-1990/.

6. *Cambridge Dictionary*, s.v. "worry," accessed May 24, 2020, https://dictionary.cambridge.org/dictionary/english/worry.

7. Nancy Wilson, "The Way Out of 'Burnout,'" Desiring God, April 11, 2016, https://www.desiringgod.org/articles/the-way-out-of-burnout.

8. American Psychiatric Association, *The Diagnostic and Statistical Manual of Mental Disorders* (DSM-5) (Washington, DC: American Psychiatric Association, 2013), 189.

9. Jeremy Engle, "Stress, Worry and Anxiety Are All Different. How Do You Cope With Each?," *New York Times*, March 11, 2020, https://www.nytimes.com/2020/03/11/learning/stress-worry-and-anxiety-are-all-different-how-do-you-cope-with-each.html.

10. Viktor E. Frankl, *Man's Search for Meaning* (Boston: Beacon Press, 1992), 75.

### CHAPTER 2

1. Brené Brown, interview by Bill Whitaker, "Brené Brown on Vulnerability and Courage," *60 Minutes*, March 29, 2020, https://www.cbsnews.com/news/brene-brown-cope-coronavirus-pandemic-covid-19-60-minutes-2020-03-29/.

2. "What Are Anxiety Disorders?," American Psychiatric Association, accessed May 25, 2020, https://www.psychiatry.org/patients-families/anxiety-disorders/what-are-anxiety-disorders; "About ADAA: Facts and Statistics," Anxiety and Depression Association of America, accessed May 25, 2020, https://adaa.org/about-adaa/press-room/facts-statistics.

3. Max Lucado, *Fearless: Imagine Your Life Without Fear* (Nashville: Thomas Nelson, 2009), 49.

4. Brené Brown, *Rising Strong: How the Ability to Reset Transforms the Way We Live, Love, Parent, and Lead* (New York: Random House, 2017), 64–65.

5. Laura Turner, "This Is a Good Time to Stop Fighting Anxiety," *New York Times*, March 12, 2020, https://www.nytimes.com/2020/03/12/opinion/sunday/anxiety-treatment-therapy.html.

6. Walter Anderson, *The Confidence Course: Seven Steps to Self-Fulfillment* (New York: Harper Collins, 1997), 34–35.

7. Henri J. M. Nouwen, *The Way of the Heart* (New York: HarperOne, 2009), 25.

8. A. W. Tozer, *Fiery Faith* (Camp Hill, PA: WingSpread, 2012), https://www.google.com/books/edition/Fiery_Faith/5nYYAgAAQBAJ?gbpv=1.

9. "Charles Spurgeon Quotes," BrainyQuote, accessed May 23, 2020, https://www.brainyquote.com/quotes/charles_spurgeon_132220.

10. Anderson, *The Confidence Course*, 36.

## CHAPTER 3

1. Annabelle Parr, "Let's Talk About Anxiety," The Center for Stress and Anxiety Management, September 10, 2016, https://www.csamsandiego.com/blog/tag/Bren%C3%A9+Brown.

## CHAPTER 4

1. Sophie Borland, "Doctors Are Urged Not to Hug Patients as the Comforting Embrace 'Could Easily Be Misinterpreted,'" Daily Mail, updated February 13, 2018, https://www.dailymail.co.uk/health/article-5384035/Doctors-told-not-hug-patients-case-complain.html.

2. Megan McCluskey, "The Coronavirus Outbreak Keeps Humans From Touching. Here's Why That's So Stressful," *Time*, April 10, 2020, https://time.com/5817453/coronavirus-human-touch/; Cathy Cassata, "How Touching Your Partner Can Make Both

of You Healthier," Healthline, June 19, 2018, https://
www.healthline.com/health-news/how-touching-your-
partner-can-make-both-of-you-healthier.

3. Quoted by Paula Cocozza, "No Hugging: Are We
Living Through a Crisis of Touch?," *Guardian*, March
7, 2018, https://www.theguardian.com/society/2018/
mar/07/crisis-touch-hugging-mental-health-strokes-
cuddles.

4. Cocozza, "No Hugging."

5. Tim Teeman, "Coronavirus Has Killed the Power
of Touch. How Do We Reconnect?," *Daily Beast*,
updated April 16, 2020, https://www.thedailybeast.com/
coronavirus-has-killed-the-power-of-touch-how-do-we-
reconnect.

6. Todd A. Fonseca, "The Secret Behind the Midas Touch:
The Surprising Power of Touch and Physical Contact,"
Science of People, accessed May 23, 2020, https://www.
scienceofpeople.com/touch-physical-contact/.

7. Teeman, "Coronavirus Has Killed the Power of Touch."

### CHAPTER 6

1. N. T. Wright, "Christianity Offers No Answers About
the Coronavirus. It's Not Supposed To," *Time*, updated
March 29, 2020, https://time.com/5808495/coronavirus-
christianity/.

2. Frederick Buechner, *Wishful Thinking: A Seeker's ABC*
(New York: HarperCollins, 1993), 2.

3. Philip Yancey, *Reaching for the Invisible God* (Grand
Rapids, MI: Zondervan, 2000), 69.

4. C. S. Lewis, "The Weight of Glory" (sermon, Church of
St. Mary the Virgin, Oxford, England, June 8, 1942).

5. Timothy Keller, *Walking With God Through Pain and
Suffering* (New York: Riverhead Books, 2013), 180–81.

## CHAPTER 7

1. Elisabeth Elliot, *Passion and Purity* (Grand Rapids, MI: Fleming H. Revell, 2003), 89.

## CHAPTER 8

1. Tim Keller, *The Reason for God: Belief in an Age of Skepticism* (New York: Penguin Books, 2008), 196.
2. Associated Press, "U.S. Online Alcohol Sales Jump 243% During Coronavirus Pandemic," MarketWatch, April 2, 2020, https://www.marketwatch.com/story/us-alcohol-sales-spike-during-coronavirus-outbreak-2020-04-01.
3. Amanda Taub, "A New Covid-19 Crisis: Domestic Abuse Rises Worldwide," *New York Times*, updated April 14, 2020, https://www.nytimes.com/2020/04/06/world/coronavirus-domestic-violence.html.
4. June Kelly and Tomos Morgan, "Coronavirus: Domestic Abuse Calls Up 25% Since Lockdown, Charity Says," BBC, April 6, 2020, https://www.bbc.com/news/uk-52157620.
5. Michael Kosnar and Pete Williams, "Pandemic Pushes U.S. Gun Sales to All-Time High," NBC News, April 3, 2020, https://www.nbcnews.com/politics/politics-news/pandemic-pushes-u-s-gun-sales-all-time-high-n1176451.
6. Jason Whiting, PhD, "Trapped at Home: Domestic Abuse During the Pandemic," *Psychology Today*, April 10, 2020, https://www.psychologytoday.com/us/blog/love-lies-and-conflict/202004/trapped-home-domestic-abuse-during-the-pandemic.

## CHAPTER 9

1. Derek Kidner, *Psalms 1–72*, Kidner Classic Commentaries (Downers Grove, IL: InterVarsity Press, 1973), 176.

2. B. B. Warfield, "The Emotional Life of Our Lord," accessed May 23, 2020, https://www.monergism.com/thethreshold/articles/onsite/emotionallife.html.

3. Kaylena Radcliff, "A War Story: 'There Is No Pit So Deep God's Love Is Not Deeper Still,'" *Christian Today*, June 28, 2017, https://www.christiantoday.com/article/a-war-story-there-is-no-pit-so-deep-gods-love-is-not-deeper-still/110251.htm.

4. Rick Warren, "God's Plan for Your Pain," PastorRick.com, July 11, 2018, https://pastorrick.com/gods-plan-for-your-pain/.